Eat Yo[ur]
Menta[l]

Pamela Moncrieffe

chipmunkapublishing
the mental

Pamela Moncrieffe

All rights reserved, no part of this publication may be reproduced by any means, electronic, mechanical photocopying, documentary, film or in any other format without prior written permission of the publisher.

> Published by
> Chipmunkapublishing
> PO Box 6872
> Brentwood
> Essex CM13 1ZT
> United Kingdom

http://www.chipmunkapublishing.com

Copyright © Pamela Moncrieffe 2011

Chipmunkapublishing gratefully acknowledge the support of Arts Council England.

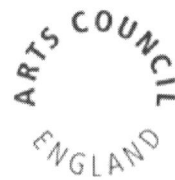

LEWISHAM LIBRARY SERVICE	
Askews & Holts	29-Oct-2013

Author Biography

Pamela Moncrieffe was born in the Caribbean Island of Jamaica in 1948.

She is a sufferer of manic depression and panic attacks, which is contained because she a firm believer in taking the prescribed medication along with a healthy lifestyle, and counseling.

Before Pamela became labeled she was a trained nurse who also had certificates in Health and Community Care, and Health and Social Care along with several other courses which she sat and was successful in.

Pamela's main interest in life is to help others where ever, and whenever she can. So writing the book Eat Yourself Mentally Fit was a great help in what she is interested in. Now Pamela's work involved her in helping individuals from all walks of life, which gives her great satisfaction.

Pamela Moncrieffe

Part 1

What to eat for mental health

Many of us are diagnosed as mentally ill people and is asking ourselves why me? Well mental illness has all the friends in this world. If you are good to all your being in time you will not encounter mental illness unless it is hereditary, if we know of our heredities in time we can some times escape it by taking care of the problem before it begins.

One of the ways of taking care of our heredities is to have thorough examination by our GP for us to be correctly diagnosed is to give accurate statement from the best of our belief, and family history. So communication is the essence of our well -being. In today's society it does not take long to form an opinion and to start a family tree. It is important to start our family tree with the natural make up of it.

We are just the branches of our family tree the trunk of the tree is what holds the truth of our make up, which is why family meetings is an essential part of our existence some of us feel embarrass at knowing we have an hereditary that could change our lives completely, and so we shun our real family and look to the ones that has a clean bill of health if it is even whilst they are young. Mental illness stem from sources of our mind and body.

The ingredients of good health is knowledge once we know what is going on in our lives we can rectify our illness. It do not mean that we should take it upon ourselves to heal our selves even though the bible said physician should heal them selves, well not all of us are physician so we should seek physician meaning do not be afraid to talk to your family doctor about your well-being.

Some times mental illness could be avoided if we took care of our strange feelings out took on things in general. Our make up is made of several different things and aspects of shield. The food we eat has everything to do with our being the right food can do so much for us, and especially our mental state. For instant if we are 3

Lacking vitamin B we can damage our selves so badly that we could become mental. Now how does the normal every day sort of person would go about sure their body consume the right amount of vitamin B that will help our mental state?

The average person eats at least 3 times a day and part of their intake should be aided with vitamin B there are several food item that holds vitamin B.

For instant malt barley and several nuts such as cashew and the fruit of the cashew the nutrients from the cashew fruit gives to the brain vital stablelising fluid and on a whole cashew fruit is a brain food, which can only be found in cashew nut and fruit it is vital because sometimes it is a deficiency that cause our mental mishap in the first place. Cashew fruit is mention because it is one of the un-thought of source of vital mental food. The cashew nut oil is different from all the other nut oils the starch in the cashew nut is vital to our vitamin B source, it is shaped like a kidney it is also of vital help to kidney complaint.

We are talking about brain feeding food, which is also known as matter food one of the most effective is olive especially the green ones it is very good for the

Eat Yourself Mentally Fit

brain it contains a special nutrient called monounsaturates

Part 2

Nutrients to help the mentally ill

Nutrient called monounsaturated which is so essential for our mental being; these are new findings are not yet elaborated on in any way that it can be an issue for our mental state. Mental health is giving cause for concern now days more and more people are becoming sufferers we would like to know that there is a menu of food, relaxation and other fundaments that we can swear by as a steadier, or a balancing for the mentally ill people. `

Mental illness is now known to start from early age and is developed into chronic state because we did not detect the symptom when they were showing signs. Why food is essential will become apparent further on in this book when saying so to develop mentally, spiritually and physically we need the right nutrient from when we were conceive.

To be born with a deficiency can some times become a life long issue with problem keeping with a special intake of a special item of nutrient. So not only adults sufferers of mental illness are to be taught to feed them selves mentally fit, but also mothers to be should be sure to take their recommended nutrient tablets, and to eat the right food right from the start of pregnancy.

Not only is it one of the brain food family it has heavenly properties for the nervous system. It depends a lot on what causes the mental instability. The first stage of rebuilding the cycle after a mental breakdown is to flourish the nervous system with good steadfast nerve food this book will give you a guideline into the areas of food that holds the nutrients, which the body needs to refurbish and restructure the cause of the breakdown.

Mental breakdown which is cause by stress need to be rebuilt with nerve food such as anything with jelly involved such as boiled cows foot made in a jelly form sea moss chicken foot any type of marrow vegetables, and one area of nerve fixing element is garlic and honey with the gizzard of a chicken grind to a powder and then be made into a combination of crushed garlic, the powder of the fowl's gizzard and the honey mix together then eat from a spoon many people add a pinch of nutmeg and often times used it as a preventative measure it is also used when the nervous breakdown happen out of the blue, and cannot be define.

A nervous could be cause from one of anything but one of the most hidden causes is infection of the nervous glands that is built up and is some times cause sudden breakdown.

When it is treated it is always with tablets, or medicine from a doctor and counselling no one as ever stop to think especially when the cause of the breakdown is classified as one of those things and nothing specific. Only nowadays a doctor will question the patient's about their eating habits, and what types of food he or she eats food has a lot to do with our mental make up.

This book is to teach us step, by step procedures into eating correct food, and eating habits that will help us to maintain good mental health. Our whole complete being has to be nutritionally fed before we can enjoy a full cycle of health. If we rob ourselves of its fortification we will have breakdown all the time, so some times when a breakdown occur and to the best of our ability we can give account of our movements we rest, we did nothing strenuous, we eat but we did not eat any of the Correct food that can correct our system but full our stomachs of what we feel comfortable with.

Here is a perfect opportunity to start catching up on what we should eat for our mental being it is not how much we eat but what we eat, and when we eat.

There is a food for every part of the body that serves their purposes well if we eat them as part of our control diet. Let us put into practice these illustrative food ideas to specify our mental strength, many of us feels that our nerves are just veins running through us, well it is no our nerves is the frame work of our being without our nerve in full working order we cannot operate as well as we should.

Nine times out of ten when we loose our nerves it affects us mentally unless it is a specific nerve then it affect us physically and even then our mentality can never be the same until it is rectified some times it can never be the same as it was be it became ill and we can only acknowledge it when our mental out look is not the same.

Our brain starts to work towards certain aspect of our being more slowly than it normally does. Which is why we should try to prevent a break down by living right and we can do so by eating right. To live right is not only to have our bath and wear posh clothe or even to keep out of trouble, the most important part of our living right process is eating the right food

Eating right is an issue we should take quite serious, serious enough to do some thing about it. We can start by taking a glance through these pages I am sure you

Eat Yourself Mentally Fit

will find out the truth about our mental feeding in some of the pages that will suit your make up.

As we all know our body needs vitamins, minerals, fat, protein, iron, carbohydrates which does not come from just one food item but from a lot of mix food items from all walks of life for our mental strength we need not only food, but also a stable home stead how ever well fed we are if we live in a hostile environment it will sop our energy and we would therefore use up much more of our natural food sources and their substances which would rob us of some times what is vital to our mentality.

So it is advisable to treat our environment as we treat what we eat. Many of us as gone through an emotional unbalancing and did not treat it with caution and so it develop into a crash unbalancing of our mental state all through lacking if guidance food also promotes our emotional state

Physical and mental performance because our bodies depends on the food composite that we intake daily if we are to live out our life span and we need not to forsake any part of our make up. Our mental state is the fundament of long life and we can assure our selves of long life span if we eat not only for our physically, but also for our mentality. Our mental health weighs heavier than our physicality because we know we must eat to live.

Eating to live is natural but our mental health some times takes a period of time before it is detected that we are neglecting our mental physique we can start caring for our mental health by experimenting on some of the food that is of natural sources, most of these foods may not be what we are accustom to but we should still try to accommodate some of these foods that are from difference sources to that which we are accustom to.

Such as tropical starch foods, vegetables and fruits they have far more vitamin D. and E than that of the foods from other sources. Here we are going to fill you in on some of the nutrients that the body needs to function mentally well on.

Our body needs all the nutrients of all the times to keep mentally fit what one area of the body needs can some times tell us what the other part is lacking. The first sign of nutrient lacking with regards to our mental health is not being able to remember our dreams and in our daily lives not being able to retain any thing from a conversation to dates and other every day issues that we should be able to remember under different circumstances.

If this start to happen we should not hesitate to start a balance plan diet after we have consulted our doctor. We should never leave it until it gets to any stage like that
Another sign is laziness, and lack of appetite one recent finding is that to suddenly become avaricious that too is a sing that our mental health is fading should that happen to us.

Whenever we are losing sleep we should check our diet sometimes we are hungry in the peak of night and cannot detect that we are hungry because of the feeling of sleepiness above all things that should drive us to a visit to the doctor the lack of sleep should take us to see our doctor.

Eat Yourself Mentally Fit

Some times the food we are eating is not right for our body make up and so it reacts on us by showing us what is wrong all these symptoms will provide evidence that we need a strict diet plan it is also telling us that we need special medicine from our doctor. Some times our bodies are crying our for special types of foods for the various mishaps that can occur in our lives our doctor are the best to discuss the symptoms with then if need be he or she can refer us to the appropriate person to help us.

Another of the symptom is a build up of energy physically the person extraordinarily energetic for a short while and then after a period of time they might suffer a laps that is because they were living on their excess energy this is when food how ever much you are eating will not help, only the help of your doctor will be of any use. Our excess energy from the nutrients we eat should be left in our body to sustain us throughout.

Unless there are evidence to the meaning of the meditation if we find our selves in any way open to such evidence before we enter into meditation wee should be sure to have a seat in the bright sunlight with our face to the east where the sun rise first in the morning and in the cool of sundown sit facing west that way you shut your chromatic cycle by opening g it in the morning sit facing east where the sun rises and do not leave our selves open but shut it by repeating the process sitting in the cool towards the east in the evening.

The management of this process will give you evidence of a serine atmosphere so when you meditate you can travel as far as you wish because your chromo is ready for the journey. That is when the sense of the meditation but no strain on the body or the mind because you are being fed in mind body and karma so your karma, mind, and being becomes positive to your body which works for you and leave you mentality fit because you put no strain on the brain

All the procedures that are mentioned in earlier pages if you do not have a staple diet you will not enjoy one minute of all those instructions. Food is such an essential part of our make up we could never be what we eat, we would not benefit from what we eat, and then how could the food that we eat work for us if it was we?

So we are our frameworks with the strong need for food to work for the up keep of our being? The that we eat and its way out of us after what does the work for the betterment of our mental system our physicality, our mind and our body is why we should never forget the essentiality of food.

Vegetable such as beet root that has its own sugar is a must because when we are pulling on our resources we need our sugar level to be on top form so apart from it high nutrients source we should eat as much beet root as possible, it works for both white cells and red cells and has a high iron level

Speaking of sugar level another form of sugar is banana another is ness berry
Jackfruit sweetsop custard apple shoran fruit all of these mention is full of iron and is good for the up keep of our mental image also the fruit of the cashew nut that is a zinc and iodine food. The summer fruits are mostly from the tropics and are exceptional the fruits are also full of vitamin A B C D E and thiamine they are most useful to our diet

Eat Yourself Mentally Fit

A mix market or a very good super market will stock all the mention fruits and those are just few others will be mention later with their mental value all the fruits mentioned are seasonal. A patient went to an acupuncturist all through the session the doctor did all she could for the patient who was suffering from severe depression the treatment was of no help. It was going through notes that the doctor called him back to the surgery the doctor found out the patient was a poor eater.

The acupuncturist put the patient on a full nourish diet and then gave him a repeat treatment the patient was almost one hundred percent well after the repeat treatment because of the full scale diet the patient was put on, if it was not that the patient was an heredity case even so his depression was controlled after the ideal diet.

So good food is so essential to our lives that to know the right type of food to eat for the many illnesses is very important my main issues are about the mental illness which is so frequent a day in the older days it was almost shameful to be mad or manic or even to have a nervous break down if wee go back into historic eating we are going to find that in those days people eat more fruits and berries than they do nowadays

Part 3

The disadvantages of fast food

Now a days there are so many man made foods that are not natural in vitamins and minerals that some times when we eat them we forget that they may not agree with our make up for body and mind nutrients. Some of us body is made to be fed with the natural sources of food and so their body rejects the man made substances without us knowing before it gets out of hand.

Our organs metabolic and mind should be fed naturally to assure us of good health all round so we can maintain quality resistance we will be left open and susceptible to all sort of system failure.

One way of assuring our selves of maintaining a quality of life is through eating fresh vegetables of all sorts and fresh fruits from all walks of life for instance if you were living in brazil you would not only eat brazil nut as your form of nut intake but you would try all other country's types of nuts. What one nut contain the other may not yet it is vital to our diet so we need to eat food from all walks of life to be sure of a channelled control diet.

Part 4 Fall backs for our body frame. It is good for our body frame to have what is called fall backs which is a built up of Nourishment in our system that acts as a rainy day resource so whenever we are weak in one source we have substitute in our body to see us through so we do not fall flat out

Eat Yourself Mentally Fit

In a way that it becomes so serious we of to have medical attention we can some times feel when we are falling below par in our body feelings and that is the time when we some times start to catch up so we should act constructively with our diet before it gets to that stage. A diet plan is easy to make, and to follow when you know what is good for the body and when you know what type of food you can digest and what type of food you like.

Some times what we like is not what is a good source of what is good for the body so some form of compromisation of to be made because it is to our own advantage that we make these compromisations one way of eating what you do not find appetizing is to find out its importance and what roll it plays in the body need resource then try to prepare it enticing and each spoon full or on the fork that you put into your mouth close your eyes and think of a healthy frame and put it slowly into your mouth think of what it is going to do for your mental state then think of your physical state then chew and swallow making sure you chew thoroughly.

To practice this you will so use to knowing what is good for you that it becomes habitual and fun. So forming a habit of good healthy eating can help us in many ways especially in our mental state vitamin and minerals are so vital to our mental health because our organs and frame work depends on our nerve and brain we of to feed these essential parts for our mentality to work and behave in the right manner.

We can start to day by using planned diets that is easy for us to follow and one to suit our pocket and fit in with our every day routine it is good that in today's society we can supplement our diet with several man make foods but it is better to eat what is fresh than what is pre cooked or some time what is raw but do not have the same nourishment as thee fresh foods and vegetables.

Some of us body needs a top me up so we can supplement our intake with vitamin tablets and health foods there is a wide variety of supplemented foods not all of them can be recommended for helping to sustaining our mental health but the ones that are of help to our mental health are labelled so it is good to know which of them is for us.

It is better to be sustained in a way that when symptoms that are contrary to how we should feel starts we will have an idea of what is going on we should never leave our selves to this theory but many of us forget our mental state some times until it is too late if we can help it we should try to let this book help us with what is vital to the first step into helping our selves. Food is the first we should take to help us into living right and feel right to be recommended as a healthy person.

A doctor can not just look at us and tell us we are well we of to feel well in our selves by thinking right, living right, but most of all we of to do what is right for our selves for us to be classified as healthy every body knows that to feel right means that we are ticking over properly meaning our mental faculties will start reacting in co-ordination with the rest of our cycle.

If we can exercise just a few daily routine such as mild exercise to start our day with and have a breakfast first thing in the morning starting with barley and dried fruits semi skimmed milk or fruit juice it should make a lot of difference if we exercise this routinely, and we should have at least one teaspoon full of honey or more

Eat Yourself Mentally Fit

or brown sugar if we are allowed sugar in our drink every day

Part 5

Ridding the self of unwanted feelings

Some of us first thing in the morning are very sluggish when that creeps in and we can not shake it with mild exercise or the usual stretch then a spoonful of glucose is advisable just so that we do not live on our reserve energy for too long we need as much reserve energy as possible especially those that helps the red cells, and the white cells and our nerve cells.

A doctor should be contacted if you have taken all the procedures and you still can not shake the dull sluggish feeling over a period of time. It may mean there is a soon break down around the corner so the safest precaution is to see your doctor.

Let us start knowing why our mental health is as much an entitlement to the food we eat as any other part of our being or our framework. We are going to make known dominant food that we should eat for our mentality to behave as it should for us to be safe from break down or mental mishap.

The menu for mental fitness the relaxation there are many ways of relaxation in meditation it is very good and healthy to be able to relax. You can actually strengthen your mind and mental faculty by relaxing every part of your being without meditation, to empty the mind you of to try to forget every thing. To put yourself into a comfortable posture you should wearing loose soft clothing some times depend on your living situation you should relax in the nude.

Eat Yourself Mentally Fit

Try to be sure that the place, room or house is clean and is of a pleasing aroma it is also advisable to make the odour of the place you are going to relax in is as natural as possible and in one half of the relaxation the room should be very lighted, and in the other half the room should be as dark as you can possible accommodate it. Then complete silence without sound in the lighted room.

In the dark room music that is just sound instead of words smooth and relaxing to energise the karma, whilst the mind sends energy to the mind and body which will account for all that you have emptied to reach a complete relaxation mood.

Once you get into the fundament of accurate relaxation it is time to move forward to actual meditation it is good to know what the meditation is about so the right mood can be set to meet the rhythm for instance if your meditation is about health you should have slow airy music, if it is for spiritual purposes then the stiller the atmosphere the better, because you will be able to reach further about the situation.

For health you want to know you can suppress obstacles and also that you can use your mind not under pressure but that you can come close to some things and pay attention to what really is at hand. Such focusing on the immediate issue forming your mental pattern swaying in and out of moods until with the music you reach the right mode to transcend leaving the almost hush music going into a pattern of echoed stillness.

By now you should be able to settle to reach the criteria you are well on your way to master your meditation techniques and so making a combination of relaxation and meditation and relaxation to suit and strengthen your mental pattern.

A menu of rightness is so essential for our well being in order to benefit our mental health. One of the first step is to listen to our selves the other is being truthful to our selves by being able to accept what seems odd in what we listen to even in our attitude we should look for changes extreme or mild it is essential that we watch our selves just as how we listen to our selves.

In all this not eating right, and at the right time and most importantly eating the right foods. If we do not bad habits can arise which will make us become very irritable with almost a label of being miserable which is when it is important that we take notice of our moods because all these changes are cause by the lacking of the right nutrient some times even listening to someone, or using the right meditation or relaxation can be seeing as mental foods. All these steps will nourish our mentality.

A lot of time we would go out of our way to catch up on a food that is recommended for this but if we were to be careful in our eating and eat correct foods all round it would solve quite a lot of our every day problems in every way. So let us catch up on some of the food we should be eating and why as part of our every day diet.

We should start any sort of reference diet, or eating plan with a main course because even though all food that nourishes is important to our bodies a main course is the most important as breakfast is the most important meal of the day. So for a balance main course for the average person we would commence with one or two mouth full of water. Then potatoes, which apart from the

Eat Yourself Mentally Fit

protein and other nutrients we should find it useful its potassium especial to eat the potatoes with the skin on it so be sure to wash the potatoes clean before cooking and keep it warm when serving.

One of the other important food is the root vegetable carrot again to be wash thoroughly clean before cooking and should not be peeled it should be cooked in the skin and should be eaten with the skin and should be served warm when cooked it is high in zinc and iodine we some times forget zinc and its importance carrot along with parsnip and beet root.

Findings about the beetroot eaten with the skin is especially good for the blood to eat vegetable and fruits in their skin that are rich in potassium and zinc enrich the blood with substances which is vital to our nerve all the items mentioned is vital to our nervous system and is a substance source to our being and is also very cheap to obtain they are always in season other known foods that helps the mentality are brown, and white rice, and also sweet potatoes again to be eaten in its skin after cooking sweet potatoes are high in iron, potassium and oxide and magnesium, magnesium prevents unnecessary fluids from building up and preventing the body from retaining bad fluids.

Part 6

Vegetables that are important to our mental health

Swede as a vegetable should be eaten as a staple food it is the best among the root vegetables oxide potassium iron and protein are the benefits from eating Swede in its skin again it should be washed thoroughly before cooking one way of making sure that you eat the skin of the Swede is to grater it, there are so many different dishes that can be made from it.

Swede fritters is quite appetising and is made with any sea food along with any other vegetables you may feel to add the thing is with Swede you hardly need any salt whatsoever especially when you blend it with other sources later on in this book you will find recipes that I know will entice you.

Many people do not like to eat Swede because of its taste well eating Swede should be taken seriously because is treated as a nerve feeding food because of its importance to our body and its high iron contexts.

Let us include in some very important vegetables beat root spinach Callao winter cabbage artichoke okras broccoli carrot chocho cucumber quash parsnip pumpkin Swede onions shallots spring onion celery garlic Brussels sprouts Chinese chow.

There are vegetables that are a must if we are to maintain a culture full balance to help the in take that will help us all through our expected intake to assure us of a healthy balance diet the nutritional values of all these vegetables will be found further on in this book.

Eat Yourself Mentally Fit

Vegetables are an essential part of every body's diet but especially for those of us who are hoping to maintain a healthy mental life. We should eat for the whole complete system of our body that way the functioning of the benefit that we receive from what we eat would have balance us and so whenever some thing is going wrong in our make up it would have been able to be detected easily or without any trouble in stead of finding out that we lacking something that could have been the cause. It is a case of preventing is better than having it to cure.

Part 7

Specific foods for mental health

Let us specific ate on a few of the nutrients that we should try our best to see to it that we eat food that is enrich with, for our mental health, iodine is one of the most important of nutrient that we should have daily intake of it influences our thyroid glands to stay healthy and so that we can develop good mental health in young or old people. It is important because lacking of iodine is some times why we develop stress that leads to serious mental break down.

The symptoms of lacking of iodine are lacking of energy constipation and severe stressful feeling. So to ensure that we do not become ill in those capacity, we should eat a lot of fish sea weed back up with un-skimmed milk cheese and jelly to feel fit and safe from mental fatigue these however are just a few of the things that we should eat to assure our selves of our iodine and they are easy to get from any market or supermarket. When our thyroid glands are under active it is as bad as when it is over active and can some times cause us to be stress beyond repair and that is when we of to rely on medication so let us promise our selves to be sure of our intake of iodine.

Iodine is an essentiality to our lives lacking of it will cause mental defect many of us many of us did not know that many people become stress whenever they are constipated well it is a well know fact so whenever we find our selves constipated in a repeated way if we are sure that we are eating foods that contain iodine then we should without fail contact our GP.

Eat Yourself Mentally Fit

We are not just thinking of being able to do number two but to assure ourselves of being topped up with our iodine how GP is best inform of how often we eat iodine if constipation occurs we should not ignore it if we have the feeling of being lazy lacking of appetite should you be opt on the subject then the first thing you would do is to detect the thyroid glands bulging below the chin and around the neck.

Some times if we are inactive we may not find a swelling but an irritable. Sluggish feeling, and so stress creeps in either way it is a serious complaint which
Leads to all sorts of mental illness so one of the preventatives is iodine which can be receive from eating the items mentioned earlier on and if we use salt in our iodine cure method we should use sea salt and bear in mind that herring fish is one of the most important when filling up on your iodine.

See weed is very rich in iodine there are several plants and herbs which can give us a source of iodine which will be categorise further on in this book. One of the other important mental health nutrients is zinc it is as important as any of the other nutrient source it is important that our body gets a full source of zinc it acts like a shield to our immune system and therefore should be taken as a serious part of our diet. Yeast which we know is in bread especially brown bread and also all form of yoghurt drinks will fill the source of zinc to eat a good amount of bread is good because it holds more than just yeast in the since of goodness.

Our most important nutrient need is iron we must have the right amount of iron to function correctively but I must quote we need all the nutrients there are in our body to live a healthy life. We should never eat without acknowledging that a source of iron is intermingled in whatever food we are eating unless you know for sure that you have deficiency of a particular type of vitamin or mineral and is topping up on it especially.

A source of iron can be found in beet root ripe banana ripe plantain and one food that is hardly spoken of is dasheen a root tuba that is grown in the tropics but should not be ignore when we are fighting to keep mentally fit. It is prepared just as you would a potato but it must be peeled the skin cannot be eaten. The dasheen is high in potassium and the type of starch that the body needs.

The starch from dasheen is like jell teen or aspic Jelly that is very good for our mental frame. Dasheen starch source is cured by the time it reaches the store for severe cases d given to be eaten of any form of nerve break down the dasheen should be dug from the grown and cook immediately and given to be eaten with good olive butter. It is especially a soup food and should be treated as part of the vegetable to any soup it will help to strengthen vital parts of the body that some times interact with our mental well being as mentioned earlier on we need to eat every thing in proportion if we are to maintain a viable health programme to enrich our lives to meet its essential needs.

On the topic of mineral roll we should also cook our meals with essential herb the surprising thing is that some herbs has more minerals and useful health given properties than even the food we praise and eat much of.

So to ensure we do not loose out a few of the important herbs will be mentioned over leaf. As we

Eat Yourself Mentally Fit

carry on with another healthy food property is oats it is full of goodness and can also help to heal the nerves.

Part 8

The Sarah Jenkins story

Right after a breakdown Sarah Jenkins started to eat raw oats and fund that she stopped speaking to herself and could hold her cup in her hand with her cup of tea as hot as she likes it. Where as before she took to eating raw oats she shakes a lot and talks to herself she swore by the oats porridge and the actual raw oats. She still takes medication given to her by her doctor but had not it been for the raw oats she started eating she do not feel she would be able to get through each day the way she does.

Here is the recipe Sarah used half a cup of raw oats quarter of a teaspoonful of nutmeg just over half of a pint of milk or your needed quantity of milk two table spoonful of good honey or brown sugar, or even glucose treat as you would a bowl of cereal and then eat.

This is a sworn recipe used by Sarah who suffered a mental break down and started eating the raw oats and got better in her mannerism and characteristics. It should eaten as a preventative method and not wait for a breakdown to start eating it.

As minerals are associated with light greatly our body needs it or it will be like us searching i9n the dark to find our way and that is how we will feel if we allow our body to become lacking of mineral it is well associated with hardness and so it is linked with iron the two are a combination and is high priority in our diet to ensure a sound mentality.

Eat Yourself Mentally Fit

A recipe for our mental state is selenium it helps our red cell if it is lacking in our body we will know because we will start doubting our self. The next is copper our body needs copper to help settle all the other nutrients so we can act consciously and calm so you see it has every thing to do with our mental health. Copper is found in this tropical fruit above all the fruits the jackfruit, although it is a fruit the seed can be cooked and then eaten, it can also be roasted then it is shelled and then be eaten with sea salt and olive butter it is full of nutrients.

The sop of the jackfruit is sweet and is filled with iron, iodine vitamin c the colour is yellow which create a calm while the seed is full of protein iodine zinc iron and phosphate the seed of the jackfruit can be eaten as food it holds other nourishing properties which is yet to be endorse.

The aim of this book is to remind us at all times that our mental state is the fundament of our well being and therefore should be taken seriously, and treated with the outmost importance these food items are a must on our plates one writer said we are what we eat and another writer said what we eat makes us what we are. Could it be that food is what we can lean on at all time?

We eat to live so to lean on food is most accepted food is not life but it saves life which is why we can always lean on it to live. A nice recipe is acke and salt fish now many people heard of ackee but do not know of its medicinal and nutritional values ackee is yellow in colour and as you know yellow is a mental tint and is use for calming situation well so is ackee when it is cooked properly it holds iron zinc iodine and potassium it is high in phosphorous all that with its accomplishment of fish and the many vegetables that can be added for serving makes it a high priority food item.

There are several types of salt fish of which all of them are rich in kelp iodine and iron protein and calcium all of these mentioned nutrients is good for our mental well being it means that we must assure our selves of eating plenty of the mentioned to store in our nutrient bank that is in our body. It do not mean that we should eat in one go a wad of these things, but to make sure that we eat them as part of our diet in proportion.

Lobster, prawn, shrimp, and crayfish I must state that crayfish is one of the shell fish we hardly hear about apart from it being a fresh water shell fish it is a sweet and tasty shell fish and is as fortified in nutrient as any other all the mentioned are well recommended source of kelp and other nutrients and should be eaten as part of our control diet source they are mentioned because they can easily be got.

Further on in this boob you will find detailed outline of all the mentioned food items usefulness and nutritional value. So let us prolong the fundaments of how to stay entirely healthy to maintain a strong and healthy mental stability. Let me mention some of the tropical fish, which good supermarkets have in stock or the local fishmonger so we can assure our selves of stocking up on them.

Bull head, mud eel, keteh keteh, goat fish flying fish and grouper, tallapong snapper gargle eye these are just a few of the fish because they are from the tropics they are high in vitamin E apart from it full fortification as other fish. One of the fish that is a must is trout; river or sea trout are closely guarded on the tropical Islands.

Eat Yourself Mentally Fit

It is only now a days the mix market sells them because of their nutritional values those who knows of their values ask fish monger specifically for them instead of buying them at random. A once in a while top me up was about a dozen keteh keteh a medium size cho cho a large carrot and a turnip with about three fingers of young green bananas and a hand full of fresh sea weed a sweet pepper and a small piece of hot pepper onion shellot spring onion sealt salt to taste a table spoon of butter.

You cut everything very thin and bring them to the boil without the fish until the vegetables are almost cook then you lay the fish on top of the other ingredients mind you please remember that according to the amount of people you are cooking for you stipulate the water that you use to cook it you must remove the fish or the bones from the soup in order to enjoy the top me up oh and do not forget a couple of ripe tomatoes to add to its richness. If you cannot get keteh keteh then by all means use salmon head the salmon head is very strong and rich in valuable nutrients, which can act as the keteh keteh would.

The vegetables do not take long to cook and as we know we should never over cook vegetable. The fish should be cooked thoroughly until the flesh leaves the bones you then spoon out the bones that can be seen, then add the rest of the ingredients to bring to the boil stir slowly as though you are mixing every thing together the butter should be stirred in until it is dissolved this is a seriously potent tonic known as the pick me upper.

In case children are participating in the eating of this tonic you strain the soup before adding the vegetables to ensure safe swallowing without bones sticking at the throat. With the salmon head you need not strain the soup because it only has straightforward bones. The fresh sea weed should be place on top of the almost cooked ready to serve ingredients, but if the sea weed is dried it should be put in the pot firstly whether you are going to strain it or not the salmon head is potent in goodness and can be used instead of any other fish.

Cook this every once in a while and our omega three is assured not only will we be helping our selves mentally by eating a lot of fish helps the heart to be steady. Another way of making up perk me ups is by using the Jamaican crackers you get three salmon head and wash them thoroughly place them into a pot with four pints of water and a small cup of barley leave them to cook until the flesh of the salmon is soft enough to have the bones remove from the pot, by then the liquid would have boiled down to at leas two pints of water you then add half a dozen shallot three or four spring onions two cloves of garlic half of sweet pepper a pinch of black pepper half a dozen Jamaican crackers you cover tightly and simmer for seven minutes.

On each bowl you put a small knob of butter then you add the prepared ingredients and serve immediately many people grater a small carrot and sprinkle over the prepared dish this is an all round nourishment dish suitable for older people.

To prepare a pick me up for ado lessons who are the most prone to small break down that if is not taken in consideration can turn into real mental problem on like old people they are also prone to infection. So to crush a generous amount of garlic two or three cloves a generous amount of spring onion a hand full of shallot a sprig of thyme half a medium Swede sliced very thin you then bring to the boil for ten minutes you cut at least two pounds of salmon fillet grate one pound of potatoes preferable red bring to the boil add a generous amount of olive butter a pinch of sea salt to taste simmer for five minutes then leave to cool and feed the child with the prepared soup as often as possible to help their boisterous behaviour, which some times is the beginning of an uncontrollable attitude unless it is detected and treated before it gets out of hand where medication is the common answer we can avoid all this if we pay attention to our children, and our selves to know that the mind do not just blow it starts from some where let us be there to detect the signs, so we can use these useful methods to help any un-natural situation we can use food as a booster method to alleviate stress, emotional, mental and even spiritually. Tablets is always the method that we turn to when prescribe by our doctor but nothing can beat the natural source.

The mentioned recipe is to the lacking of vital nutrients these ingredient holds apart from the every day diet we should always treat our body to top ups so we can store nutrient for healthy living it should be seen as a best dress, best shoes sort of a thing we can never tell when we are going to of to call on our resources.

Our body need nourishment every day because our mental health depends on us if we do not show our selves that we are in control of our complete being then that part will control us when that happen is when talking to our selves and acting strange and not responding to our every day sort of attitude as we should creeps in and all because the responsibility of making sure our diet is correct and consist of all the right nutrient.

The cause of mental break down can only be cause of lacking of the right food, emotional problems, and if we are not ready to enter into deep spiritualism or if we task our selves too much. It helps tremendously if we eat correctly so the nervous system in our body function correctly. If a break down happen our side those known zone it can be detected quickly so the right diagnosis can be made.

The reason for the many methods other than foods that are explained is to show us that our body rely on every thing that is good to fulfil our being needs and so those of us who have heredities can get detected and so be diagnose in time before it becomes chronic. Let us get into some ideal foods easy to get hold of and easy to prepare thank God for import and export we can purchase every thing that is about to be mentioned in this book and every thing that is already mentioned.

Please quote that this is not a book that compels you to eat every thing that is recommended, but every thing that is recommended is of great value to our mental health ant the whole of our make up. I think that this is where you will admit that we some times forget our mental health when we are eating, if we would bear in mind the fact that we should treat our being as though we are pregnant, man or woman eating for two, only in this case it is rightness that matters and not quantity.

A full scale issue of what we should eat will be mentioned later on in this book let us find out step by step what we should do about creating mental food sources. For instance an egg holds every thing that a chicken is made up of and we all know what powerful nutrients we get from eating chicken we should never allow a week to go by without eating a boil egg or some of us likes it waxy. Once upon a time we well beat an egg with a pinch of nut Meg a glass of freshly squeeze orange juice some time a tot of brandy was a big pick me up.

Eat Yourself Mentally Fit

For a real tonic for the mental system a large tin of Guinness a half a pound of fresh or dried sea moss half a teaspoon full of nut meg two table spoon full of honey a half pint tub of full cream you boil the sea weed in a two pints of water bring it to the boil until it is about one pint of liquid stand it to cool or put it in the refrigerator to set it will turn into a jelly like substance you seep half the amount into a liquidiser along with the nut meg honey full cream and a half of the pint tin of Guinness you then liquidise and serve with ice or warm from the liquidiser. Depending on the amount of people you invite for the tonic night or if you have a big family then you use the remainder of the ingredients accordingly hoops forget to tell you about the eggs you add two or three eggs to the mixture before liquidising it the egg is the star of the tonic so do not forget it.

If you do not have a liquidiser you can whisk the eggs and the other ingredients into a large pot, or bowl and then ladle it as you would a punch. Mixing every thing together should give you a very frothy mixture, which is how you know it is very nourishing this concussion should be very tasty serve with crush ice In a cup, or glass should be enough to convince you to make it again for a pick me up for the mental and nervous system.

Full cream milk, or skim milk can also be added instead of cream it will not spoil the potency of the tonic make sure the eggs are from reputable retailer if you did not rear them yourself to avoid salmonella.

This is a once in a while tonic for the nerve, and for the rest of the body need thhe body also need sulphur as part of its nutrient. It would take a lifetime to name all the nutrient that the body needs to keep us safe from falling below our expected health level. So the main nutrients that are mentioned are those that would seem hard to come by and the food items that hold those nutrients are mentioned.

Our body needs more than just:

Protein
Fat
Oils
Carbohydrates
Minerals
Vitamins
Fibre
Water

As mankind progress so is their findings on how food can help us prolong life if we are going to live longer then we need our mental faculties to be working correctively for us to enjoy full life. Another of the method that is of great help to our mental health is believe it or not is our breathing many of us do not take time to exercise breathing rhythms to send the brain the right message, our breathing also helps us retain when we retain we do not use up excess energy to try to remember, but to add to our mental faculty.

There is not any one food that can solve our body need it takes all the foods to help us maintain our full sustenance of nutrient. If you are mentally ill and have it controlled and feel you should fallow the method of this book if you are a blood pressure sufferer then you must seek a nutritionist who will diagnose portion for you especially in the starchy foods such as yam potatoes dasheen pumpkin they are all good food for nutritionally but if you suffer from blood pressure you must have your diet portioned so you eat the agreed amount that is right for you.

Eat Yourself Mentally Fit

This brings us to the amount of energy we need to live feeling good within our selves this varied in fat people, active people, people who are born lazy, and people who are made inactive because of ill health.

Our body needs 15000KJ per day that amount especially if you are suffering from a mental breakdown or recovering in other words place on medication to balance and control the illness the thought of being mentally ill starts off a pattern of anxiety and as we know anxiety sops energy because the mind is working non stop when anxiety arose. Then again if the mental illness is what is called silent madness even then we use up more energy because we then rest on our reserve energy that we build up.

This amount of energy need that is mentioned is especially for mentally ill people. For a normal person using this method to prevent a break down then the amount of body energy per day that is needed is about 11 KJ if they are active men they need 13 KJ, and for women 12KJ is needed per day when they are truly active. Those who are retired getting on in age need less energy they are slower than young active people so they need about 9KJ per day that amount will balance each individual that are retired.

That recommended energy need for each day is for adults. For children who are super active age 5 to 11 years of age body need of energy is 8KJ when they are boisterous, calm and not so playful children's need is 7KJ per day and can still enjoy healthy lives. It varied in girls during the monthly period up to 9KJ per day is advisable so they can still keep their reserve energy in tact because girls lose their appetite during their period.

Boy need up to 12KJ per day if they are age 12 to 15, and again young men age 16 to 19 need up to 13KJ per day if they are fully active if they are not active then their daily energy need is 10KJ. For a office worker who is manic or suffer from stress they need the maximum amount of body energy to see them through and to keep them going.

Part 9

A recommended amount of our salt intake

An adult should eat no more than 4to 5 grams of sea salt per day and children half that amount. We should also bear in mind that there is no one food item that can specify a mental break down it takes all sorts of food to help get any person back on their feet unless the cause unless the cause of the break down is specified, and diagnosed then with medicine and the prescribed food the person may recover in other words with a proper diagnosis because of known facts about the break down or the cause of the mental illness we must not take our diet for granted we must also rely on a proper diagnosis.

Here is not forgetting that people suffering from mental illness some times do become pregnant so the pregnant woman body energy need is 12KJ per day and a woman who is mentally and have a baby see fit to breast feed then their daily body need of energy is 13KJ per day. The extra energy is to fill the gap because mentally ill people need more energy than the normal person because they are using up energy subconsciously also. So it is a separate amount of energy that is needed to cope with being mental to live a control balance life.

We should try to eat a balance diet at all times at all times and if it is not possible for to eat a balance diet at all times then we should make up for it whenever we can not only in quantity, but in quality vegetables, herbs, foods, and fruits that holds the vital nutrients that the body needs. It stem from lacking of iron to the very minimal of nutrients in the body for us to fall rapidly from good health to poor health.

We have avoided an important issue in all what we are doing we know about stress and some of us even know how to cope with stress, but very few of us as ever been diagnose that our stress is caused by lacking of the right nutrient in our body. This stress is called psychological stress all unknown to us when it strike our only way of knowing is when we start to take note of our action and include the food we eat and when we eat.

Some people use stress as though they are playing Russ eon roulette with their being well no stress is good for the alterative people who are assertive and is balanced they can detect stress and nine out of ten times deal with it, because they have their stress management worked out and can deal with amicably.

Those of us who are less fortunate and live in a categorise standard, and is poor educational status should stay well away from stressful situation because it can be e easily gets out of hand.

When we are speceficating we should also know that excessiveness in our diet can cause trouble, and in-excessiveness can also cause trouble things such as sugar and starch is what we should eat in measured portions.

For instance many of us own a blender, which we use to juice fruits when we juice the fruits we should always use the flesh or the sop of the fruits which some time is called residues after the juice is extracted, that will enable us to get all the goodness such as the pectin because juices the pectin is harden and is left in the `sop. That is why the sop of orange, apple, grapes, peach, apricot in fact every fruit that is juice for marketing a substance of to be used in it to allow the pectin to filter also in the fluid that is the industrial measure, but if we are juicing fruits at home then we should not take it for granted that we are getting one hundred percent of the fruit.

To ensure that we get all the nourishment that the fruit carries we should eat the whole complete fruit or if we juice them we should eat the sops make sure that we eat the sop, segment, or fleshy part that is left after juicing them.

Some times the way the fruit, vegetables, or food sources ie herbs are grown gives us a reason to list our food before relying solely on it. If it was possible for organically grown food and vegetables and herbs to be our source it would solve many fears and problems. Many people are made up different from others and so our body absorbency reacts differently to source such as food and water and air.

Many unsolved medical cases will of to be given a review into the food we eat, and the water we drink and our oxygen intake for instant the more polluted the area the more dense the air and so it can cause lung decongestion where a person of to fight through the density with their lung paying the price of society responsibility.

So is our food fertiliser that is use for the help of food growth can give off a chemical reaction in a person's body who is not yet discovered that they are sensitive to a chemical in the food they eat. Nine out of ten times allergy is not from the food it self, but from some thing it is carrying from the growth so to eat organically is well advised.

It can help to alleviate the pressure of not knowing what causes what. In organically grown foods if an allergy occurs it is a food allergy and not the substance it was mannoured with or the substance that was used to help promote more for what it is worth known a fertiliser.

There should be a test of this sort but unfortunately there is no known test of this sort, but to eat and then wait for the reaction. Some times it is too late after eating the food that is bad for us over a period of time apart from terrible physically ill it some times result into us being diagnose mad, because from hypoactive to acute stress situation to madness whether we where mentally ill or not.

We need food that carries mental tint, such as the colour red, yellow, orange, purple white peach, and blue so we should try as much as possible to eat food that are those colours to calm us and to do other helpful things to our mental state.

As you know it is not only our mental state that will be at stake if we are mal fed our whole complete is to be nourish in order for us to perform mentally spiritually emotionally and physically correct. So let us take care of our all and at the same time try to correct and keep right what could go wrong if we get careless with our diet.

Let me state again there are a lot of step that can be taken to maintain a quality of life with every thing and every part of our body care to insure a perfect life. After all now a days there is longer life to living long we of to participate in what is right for our being and it starts with good food every part of our being is important.

Eat Yourself Mentally Fit

Especially if we would like to make an impression in society, we of to start with the right mental attitude to abstain and maintain that we of to take care of our every part.

It is a job in it self to keep in the right mental attitude and to keep our self in the right mental frame. The method used can be so varied such as yoga meditation relaxation spiritual awareness and emotional balancing. We of to be strong all round to maintain the full cycle.
Part 9 Chart for our wellbeing.

There are so many measures to reach these criteria if we are not mindful of our welfare so let us work out a measure of mindful tact on our own behalf firstly we should all have a chart of our well being care status that way we will work towards living up to its expectation a lot of us would have had a constant reminder of what is on the list of priority in our life. That way we will be on the right tract to a better assured life of living all round.

We some times feel if we are stress prone, or manic or is sick mentally we cannot get the illness controlled enough to enjoy life but that is not true, mental illness can be controlled it depends on the density of the illness how far gone the illness is every one of us at one time or another in our lives as suffered stress have a near break down or let something emotional get out of hand.

How often we feel offish and buckle down to a check up at the doctor or truly feed our selves emotionally, physically, spiritually, and socially by loving our selves enough to identify those needs and be astute enough to see to it that these needs are met but we can only be astute in those areas if we are constructive enough to identify when it is time for caring about ourselves in the operative way.

For us to operate with cousion in order for us to be right inside out it takes a method known as the self-regime man in other words all else is secondary to our lives we are number one mind body and soul the vital word is respect we must not lose respect of our selves in or to be independent of short falls that could easily bring us into lacking of what we need for our whole being to remain respectfully right, or well.

One of the most important state of our well being is our social life it is apart of our affair and needs types of feeding or wee will find our selves with drawn from society and find it hard to intermingle then we are left open and susceptible to self pity relying too much on our self until it becomes an emotional problem.

So we need to take in account our whole being from food to our intermingling and believe it or not when we eat good food we will feel good about our selves and want to share the joys of good health with others in a round about way to socialise is like eating good food the company you form is like the way the way the food is cooked and then the enjoyment is a matter of taste.

To feed our selves mentally well we of to include all that it takes to give us a smile some thing to reflect upon like a nice healthy dinner.

We all know that children can also become mentally ill. When this occur nine out of ten times it is either an heredity or many mothers do not know that when they are breast feeding they should be stress free because the baby will drink emotional milk instead of balanced breast milk.

Eat Yourself Mentally Fit

It is known that anxiety fluid is what baby drinks from the mother if their mother is upset when breast feeding nothing is worst than emotional milk it act like a clock it tick over an d over but hit at the same thing until it makes itself clear. Some time the milk in mother stops if the mother gets terrible emotional it is like an electrical shock the reaction delays until the current is charged, then a reaction visible or known.

So to ensure that a child is fed balanced breast milk the mother should ensure calm in their being for the milk to flow as milk instead of unbalanced fluid which can cause prolong mental unbalancing in children as they grow. The signs are hypo activeness autism sometimes even blatant mental disposition because they drink the bad useless fluid that should be express and throw away, then after the situation is settled the true milk can be given. In other words avoid a quarrel, stressful situation or a shock of any kind if you are breastfeeding if you have an unsure situation at home try to give your child milk from a bottle. Children who slow in speaking walking and learning apart from a thousand other reason mothers who fret a lot can actually harm their children by breast-feeding the rhythm that the milk is made up of is affected by the mother who is troubled.

Such situation such situation can also cause distraction as he or she grows it can even sometimes stunt their growth it also affect their behaviour pattern and also their learning pattern which is why the disorder is labelled distraction the anxiety pattern in children comes from actual shock or harm done directly to the actual child.

Let us look at ways that we can deter harmful situation that we can cause our children by avoiding the what will cause the harm what this feeding is aiming to do is to show mothers who have disturb children just what causes them to be disturb and ways to avoid the problem because from a disturb child to a really mentally ill adult.

Part 10

Away to be assured of sound mentality

Many things can cause a person to be labelled disturb nine out of ten times the lacking of the right food by the mother from before the child was born the breast milk is the child's food while they are at that young age oh bless progress and the many alternatives that is available now a days. Even in having the many different milks that babies can be given at birth, breast milk is still the best even if the milk is to be express from the breast to a bottle to feed the child so the child become clematises to food that is necessary for them in later years through what the mother eat which makes up the milk.

Feeding the baby that way helps to alleviate eating disorder in the child as they develop. For the baby's sake no slimming should not take place while a mother is breast feeding if this happen you will find that the children involved whilst growing up will be fretful, and slow because of the break down of energy that is lost through the less eating and sometimes a prep up certain types of food that we may become complacent with.

In eating this way it gives the child a variety of indulgency disposition from a hat psychological point of view and providing the illness namely mental disturbance is not heredity then you would be sure to be building up a resistance level in you child by eating the right food to breast feed it back to the child.

Good food eaten by a mother who is breast feeding not only sustain the child but help to maintain a stable mental balance in later years such years as when they start school, and mixing with other children. Many times the school to parents is that the child is with drawn from other children. That detection if the home life is free from abuse is either if the child was breastfed or was not given the right types of food as an introduction when they start on solid or the mother did not eat the right food whilst she was carrying the child or whilst she was breast feeding.

One of the most important in children is to introduce different types of food sources that holds nutrients the body can rely on for sustenance. If you wait too long before giving the child the type of food that matters if the child is lacking the right nutrient and can be of great destruction to their physical, emotional, and mental health the lacking of important can be very harmful to children and adult alike.

Especially when the child of to rely on one source some times only energy they live on until it is found out some times it is far too late to rectify completely and so end up with a sick situation that of to be maintain and control none of us like that situation so let us try to prevent all those issues by starting to take more notice of our eating behaviour and pattern especially mothers to be.

The phrase eating for two is very important and should be taken seriously. It is not the amount that is eaten but the type of food that is eaten for instant when a woman is pregnant she should think of the child's well being. In the sense of physical emotional and mental welfare their spiritual well being is by adoption or self indulgence so a visit to the nutritionist is a good idea.

To indulge in reading which is good for a mother to get versed up on what food is very necessary for both mother and baby. One important issue is that to adopt a principal of reading will open the appetite and because of what is read if you pick a book on nutrition you would know exactly what to eat and that is how the average person ensure that both them and their children eat right, and in the case of a pregnant woman to read whilst pregnant will give them an intellectual karma and rhythm which is good for the baby whilst still in the womb.

A lot of our health problem started from we were in the womb, that is why break through now a days is helping us a great deal to identify our heredities and so it can be remedied before we are left with it feeling it is something that as to remain with us.

All these efforts to reach these factors help us mentally and spiritually whilst our physical status is visible and so can be rectified at any short notice emotionally things of to go wrong emotionally and spiritually before it can affect us mentally.

Some times we feel emotionally and physically fit and think that our mental health is in good state, but it is by paying attention to our well being why we even some times detect that some thing that seem right is oh so wrong to be in the right is to start and it is from a foetus to a child and the growing up if the right attitude is applied to our well being that a full bill of health can be endorse on our behalf.

When we grow up and in one time or another the doctor gives us a clean bill of health we owe so much to our parents mothers especially. Then it is up to us to continue to keep well by following what our parents or guardian do to ensure us being healthy. So communication is essential at this stage in our lives if only to know where we are at with our heredities.

So if along the way we have adopted any illness we can tackle it before it gets out of hand. On a whole it do not take long to find out if we are in good health, because what do not apply will fight against what is right in our body, and because we are healthy we will recognise the signs. That is when detecting what is wrong is easy.

Instead of having to probe all over our physical, and emotional being especially if what is wrong is of a mental nature. That is when our psychological being can never rest, nine out of ten times that area is where is to be blamed for what is wrong so our mental state is question.

This feeding should help to give us an idea of what mental feeding is about, so let us exercise it. When we read we are exercising mental feeding, when we communicate we are exercising mental feeding when we meditate we are exercising mental feeding but all this of to be on a constructive level. One way of knowing whether our argument is constructive is to recognise the response of others that we are communicating with.

It is also advisable to carry out these objectivities with complete strangers who do not know your characteristic so their response can be treated as impartial

In children it is easy to recognise if they are backward in any way because they depends solely on parents or guardian for their sustenance if we are going to detect any form of in-normalities cause through lacking of the right food from their eating habits or through the lacking of the right food when they were conceive meaning the mother not eating the right while they were carrying the child. This detection can be identified through the child slow in speech and also walking even to comprehend they have a slow uptake.

As the cows milk holds vital nutrients coming from what they eat and if the cow itself is healthy so is the milk so is the mother of any child that is breast fed breast feeding is not just for bonding but for rhythmical transferring vital issues which is necessary for the child's well being as well as bonding and it all have something to do with the child's growth from in the womb to baby, to infant, to toddler to ado lesson into young adult.

That is how heredities are known from the mere lacking of nutrients from the child was in the womb these are vital statements which are identified in several of the cases of mental illness in boys and girls. After the age of eighteen it is highly unlikely that we can blame mental illness on what the mother was lacking when she was carrying the child in other words when she was pregnant.

So any detection should be when the child was toddler or early teen after that it is true that they have form have form their own characteristics and in such away that if they them selves did not eat the necessary foods it is because unlike in the womb it was not given to them as a growing child.

Many of us eating habits are spoilt through our parents not because they could not afford the food that is necessary but take it for granted that since they do not like certain food the whole complete family should go without it.

Well it should not be so some children has never heard of herbs and many of the minerals that is good for them because parents have not the time to disgust food with their children. They of to wait until they are old to either read about the real good food that they should eat or wait until they can prepare it for them selves they make do with the basics.

Many of the time we would put those situation down to people of the third world countries but it is not so, in the third world country there are vital herbs, vegetables and food in general even fruits that we would laugh at which holds vital source of nutrients you would find in places that are lacking aviation and suffering heavy drought but on a whole these countries when the harvest is in have some of the very best nutritional foods, and because of tradition the whole complete family is well fed at a early age.

It is us in the western world that pick and chose in such a way that some times we chose what is bad for us a packet of crisp instead of an apple a cup a tea with two sugars instead of a cup of mint tea with a teaspoonful of honey or glucose sugar instead of eight pints of top water we should try four pints of top water and four pints of mineral water.

That way our data is sure to work for fat and impurities mineral water is known to cut fat by half the fizz has a lot to do with its use it also is very good to clear the system of the body when it is carbonated it is best. Babies cannot drink carbonated water so their water should be boiled up until they are age three when they should be given top water so they can accumulate anti bodies to help their resistance.

Eat Yourself Mentally Fit

If the body cannot fight anti bodies that is when we need pipe water and good nutrients to build our resistance many children are sick more time than they are well until it turn into a child's lethargy cannot wake up in the mornings and wants to skip school. We do not try to find out we blame them and think that it is down right laziness. The first thing to check for is worms whenever a child is trying to take time off school and is eating picky or avariciously and sleeps a lot.

The first step that should be taken is a trip to the doctor because this can lead up to deep stress, which can very easily turn into mental depression and it all started from the body fighting anti bodies

All these summing up is to is to show us how easy it is for us to develop mental problems with us wondering where is it coming from especially when our family do not have a mental trait, it starts some times from we were in the womb and it do not of to be hereditary. So good food in the right quantity at the right time is so very much advisable. The new break through medically is endorsed by common sense and one who any one who reads this book will see truth in it

Part 11

Detecting stages of the lacking of the right food

Let us familiarise our selves with detecting stages of threat to a mental breakdown or mental illness in children which is cause through lacking of the right food.

When their immune systems are weak these are the types of illness that they may suffer, which can easily cause mental illness. Lost of appetite can cause a break down of the immune system but the lost of appetite is cause by many different reasons so let us stress on the main points.

Bad tooth laziness not being able to digest the simplest of food head aches poor eyesight hypo activeness in some cases in some cases some children just cannot eat enough they are always hungry that is when they are craving for a nutrient that they are lacking until they are given that nutrient they will go on being labelled greedy until it is found out and they are given the right food or its supplement in tablets or fluid.

So lacking of some nutrients can develop into a child going stealing from anywhere they can. When that is not what they wanted to do they are just hunting for what they cannot define it is not detected because it is not being looked at as a lacking of something that they are missing when children steal food item.

If we were to take note of what food item children who steal took from where ever they steal food from we would know how true this theory is because we would learn what they are lacking from what they are not

Eat Yourself Mentally Fit

eating so they go searching for it, it is instinct and what their psychological frame react on.

Then again children who are sufficiently fed, and is still lacking vital nutrient which is important to their well being, you will find that the parent is to be blamed especially the mother the father can only be blame if the illness mentally is hereditary and the mother can safely state that she eat right whilst she was carrying the child, and the hereditary is not from her

In most cases the mother is blame. In pregnancy the hormone changes can cause all sorts of eating disorders such as soon after eating the food is out by vomiting and sometimes the morning sickness never ends so the mother becomes reliant on what makes her feel good.

Nine out of ten times what makes them feel good is not what will fortify the foetus stage the child would have still be lacking nutrient while too much of what is not good for the child have the child develop what is going to cause mental illness from that young stage

Young children get stress and some times that is where mental illness starts and if a survey of how it started should be carried out you will find that it is from the mention lacking of notice. So let us pay attention to what could spell danger long term if it is not taken in hand from an early stage

Babies who cries through out their infant age is to be investigated also many a times mothers breast fed and eat the wrong food it upset the child's stomach nine out of ten times a method of rubbing the back because the first instinct is that it might be trapped wind. Well this is so wrong the child must be given boiled water to break the acid that causes the gripe.

The feeding mother should recollect on what she might have eaten before breast feeding if it is put down to just wind and there is no way of settling the poor child
That too can have all sorts of psychological effect on the child

If you put a child who cries a lot when they were a baby up against a child of balance disposition you will find that the child who are balance smile or laugh a lot while the child you usually cries a lot is very serious, or very quiet. That is a psychological effect just like a after mask especially if it was not found what was lacking why the baby only cries even if it was only for a period of time`

This summing up to show in a round about way how young children develop mental problem from early age and how to pin point issues that are so often over looked because the child cannot really speak to say what is wrong a vase percentage of time food and lacking of the right type of food is the problem

Children and adult who do not laugh and smile a lot always end up with severe stress problem which if it is not taken seriously will develop into mental problem here are just some of the food that will help adults and children to laugh and relax to prevent stress.

These foods will be mentioned later in this book firstly these important points must be made. Mothers are warned not to drink alcohol or smoke when they are pregnant it is not only lung problem it cause or blood disorder it can derive into your child becoming mentally ill after a while so those who are venerable should stay

Eat Yourself Mentally Fit

away from alcohol and smoking also sleep enforcement aids such a liquid or tablets

Mothers should try hard as possible to get natural sleep when they are pregnant or it could leave grave mental illness on the child. Nor should a woman who are breast feeding take any sort of sleeping aid herbal supplements are advisable. Now let us get down to the type of foods to keep us smiling and laughing because we are happy with our selves

Ripe bananas
Shoran fruit
Anything with vitamin B complex
Winter cabbage
Rice
Cherries
Grapes
Red grapes
Peach
Apricots
Anything containing zinc
Iodine
Selenium
You should also go for the jack fruit
Nesberry
Star apple
Sweet sop
Sour sop
Instead of a sandwich have a bowl of good corn flakes

All these food sources are to avoid mental break down, and to fortify the nervous system. That way any weak area will be nourish to prevent break down

One of the very first symptoms of mental health is lost of appetite or over avariciousness that is when the individual is feeding on their reserve that they are made up of, when it gets to that stage it must be looked into quickly, and carefully. Please quote that the laughing foods that that are mentioned is suitable for adults and children, nursing mothers, and pregnant women.

Our nervous system also needs root foods such as cassava, pumpkin, sweet potatoes, quince, spring green cook with camomile so the infusion from the boiled spring green can also drink for a good night sleep. Although some times the goodness of then food is not mention while the food itself is evidence that it should be eaten so the most vital nourishing evidence can be mention

We should eat a lot of raw oats
All the fresh vegetables we can get to prevent depression also we should be sure of an intake of vitamin B complex. We should drink apple leaf tea and apple blossom tea keep well away from the common tea unless it is decaf instead we should have infusion of herbal teas as much as possible

Here is a menu for the prevention of depression
Raw oats
Brazil nuts
Yoghurt

Cornmeal cook for fifteen minutes and then add yoghurt glucose and a pinch of nut meg will help too keep you calm and is full of goodness. After such eating such as this a cup of camomile tea is always advisable, also if you really want some calming or a good night sleep a cup of lemon verbena with a hint of cinnamon

Eat Yourself Mentally Fit

Lacking of sleep can also cause stress so when and if this occurs you need barley water camomile tea, fennel tea, hot lime, hot lemon, and lime blossom with marjoram tea fifteen minutes before you go to bed

Many of us are hungry when we wake up at nights and find if difficult to go back to sleep. Well here is a way to ensure a all night sleep grater a piece of pumpkin big enough to full a medium size baking tin mix half a pound of stone grown flour generous amount of honey pinch of nut meg and a pinch of cinnamon 3 eggs well b eaten with the yoke one tea spoon full of lemon juice you mix all the ingredients together and grease the baking tin making sure the baking tin is big enough to hold the ingredients

Using your discretion you pre heat the oven gas mark four you then place the tin with the ingredients in and watch it periodically until it is bake like a cake. The milk and the sultanas are not mention because it is a night time food and should not be too heavy. After the pudding is baked you remove it from the oven and stand it in a cool place until it is cool and then remove it from the tin stand it on a plate. Slice at night time just before you retire for bed and eat giving it enough time to digest before you go to sleep. Treat as you would a cake

To know when the cake is bake you should wipe an eating knife clean and pearce it through the cake if it is clean after removing it from the cake then it is bake you should pierce it through several parts of the cake to make sure it is bake thoroughly

This recipe is brought about because lacking of sleep can cause stress which is the main source of depression. The lacking of the right food can cause to loose sleep and feel irritable enough to develop a fatigue. Let us try to put some practice into some genuine recipes we some times eat words to help us, now let us try some real food reading about the food we eat so we can know about it

Let us make up a dinner for laughing as we know a good laugh drives away stress and to keep smiling suppresses depression. Let us start with food for children to keep them mentally fill

Let us start off with what is healthy and also helps with their omega 3, I would state herring fish but it is highly bony and not all children are careful when eating Fish

Let me start with some fish that can be filleted such as:

Salmon
Mackerel
Sardines
Brim
Cod
Barracuda
Monk fish
Tuna, and anchovies are small fish but very oily though they cannot be filleted they are rated to be very nutritional and is recommended because the bones are very soft along with these fish advisable to cook with them for recommended value in nutrition are hemp seeds, and flax seed, and pumpkin seeds. These along with safflower seeds sesame, walnut, evening primrose, borage oil, blackcurrant seed, in cooking all these to add an egg can prove very helpful

All and every vegetables is very good for adults and children. Calcium food such as cheese milk yoghurt and

Eat Yourself Mentally Fit

many of the vegetables and herbs that is mention has their own calcium level also cereals and porridge. Many people advice against white bread to eat only brown bread is still defeating the objective, so I advice half and half if on a Monday you have white bread as toast, then by all means on a Tuesday you should have brown bread toast, that is what I feel is balanced

As with drinks pure fruit juice is a must, but once in a while because children are quite energetic they burn up calories than adults do. So to help their immune system they should once in a while be treated to a soda pop, and many children will not hear of berries, well it is so important for parent to introduce berries as you would an apple or an orange to help them mentally they need all these essentials

Many parent are told not to indulge their children to a packet of crisp, well potatoes are full of calcium and protein not forgetting other minerals and goodness. It is the salt and oil that the crisp is cooked with that is bad, to cook the equivalent to a packet of crisp in good olive oil or rape seed oil or oil of evening primrose would lesson the danger that applies to a packet of crisp that is cooked in ordinary oil or fat

A snack that is advisable is rice cake, oat meal crackers and the best a oat cake and cookie. Many parent feels it is best to give their children spaghetti instead of rice well the two are importantly essential

This brings us to essential nuts, which is a must to our diet. The part these nuts plays in our lives will show us that our whole being is to be fortified that no part of do not of to rely on the other, but has its own fortification that way we are balance

Brazil nuts for selenium
Cashew nuts for calcium, iron, and zinc
Almond nuts for calcium
Coconut for vitamin C and is also rich in potassium, phosphorus and zinc
Chest nuts carbohydrate you can eat as many as you like it is very low in fat
Walnuts and there are several different types of walnut which contain a very high level of linoliec acid which help to lower cholesterol
Hazel nuts is rich in vitamin E also peanuts are very high in vitamin E
Pecan nuts is very good for the immune and is very high in zinc to eat as much as you can is good

Let us not forget that many mental health sufferers do have other ailments, and so the foods mentioned is modified to help all the known ailments that may occur. The word mental health, do not mean that you are finish in life, if you are a sufferer it can be controlled and food is one of the safest way of controlling mental health, along with the right thinking attitude

It is true because many sufferer are very good cooks, and have an eye for good food and a taste to match the best food or the food that do good for our body. All else should be watched, a little bit of junk food every once in a while or food of contrary do not hurt, but we must not live on it but see it as a treat and keep the noted food as our dietary food

Let us catch up on some of the seeds that we so often time miss out on. They are so simple to use and do our body the world of good

Let us start with pumpkin seed which is so high in minerals such as zinc and iron and can be eaten any hour of the day and by any one. Children can eat them they are very small and easily chewed, when it is parched it is hard as peanut but un parch they are soft and moist smaller than peanuts children can enjoy them also

Sunflower seed is very good for the immune system and is very rich in vitamin E there some part of the world that swore by sunflower seed and its goodness

Sesame seed is high in calcium there are two sorts of sesame seed one sort is dark and one is very light tan in colour

Flax seed is high in omega 3 so instead of some fatty fish flax seed can be eaten for omega 3
Melon seed is very high in magnesium and in more than just traces of iron it also provide zinc and folate these are mentioned because many of us throw away our melon seeds we may ask what type of melon seed are high in these minerals, because there are so many different types of melon

All types of melon seeds are full of goodness and especially the common melon the one that is red in side and the seeds are black in colour to parch them and then grind them or mill them it is very good on cereal, and in soup and porridge or mix a table spoon full of glucose sugar to a half a pound of mill melon seed mix well and place in a clean dry jar to eat when needed. It is best place on the palm of the hand and then lick with the tongue it is full of iron and very good for building up the energy
Fennel seed is a must even if you are labelled mentally ill you should always take care and pride in your appearance, and fennel seed is just the thing to help

take care of your weight, eaten on bread, put in soup and can be use as an infusion to drink as tea

Fennel seed can be used in our gravy or in the case of obesely over weight people it can be use in your drinking water make as you would tea, it can also be seep and then infuse and can drink warm with honey for rapid weight loss

Anise seed is very good for the digestive system and can be seep and drink as a infusion
Dill seed can be use in curry to help those people who love a curry but cannot digest it after eating it
Caraway seed helps those of us who suffer from dry mouth, some times the medication that a mental ill sufferer is on can leave the mouth dry that some times a lip balm is the saviour well an infusion of caraway seed sip slowly at night for a week should help you to retain vital fluid

Let us step into some fruit that are easy to get hold of, and also is very affordable mango with its mental tint of yellow which is calming in every way it is also hig in the advisable list for blood pressure high or low its sugar helps low pressure, and its balance iron helps the high pressure. Some mental sufferer do suffer from high blood pressure caused by one thing or another
Many learned people recommend it for the remedy for high blood pressure, to peel the mango and use the skin as an infusion with a tea spoonful of honey and sip it slowly is a must it is so full of vitamin c, and it also helps to settle the stomach and gives you a sweet smelling breath
Grape fruit is full of iron that is why it is a suggested breakfast food to start us off with the right amount of iron as well as vitamin c

Eat Yourself Mentally Fit

As lemon, orange, ugly fruit, is known to be all detoxing valuable fruits ugly fruit is good for children with eating problem especially when they are picky eater the iron context opens the appetite. It acts for children and adults alike. Taking medication for mental health can either open the appetite, or have you loose your appetite, it one should loose their appetite then the ugly fruit, and the grape fruit is the answer

Lemon is or I should say is counted among the detoxing agents as one of the most powerful, it is also use as an antiseptic so cystitis sufferer after a trip to the doctor apart from what is prescribed, it is never wrong to seep a table spoonful of lemon juice in the bath water it helps the seal the complaint and dry it up

Any ailment can cause stress, but especially lacking of sleep which is why some times it is good to watch what we eat before retiring to bed. Sleep food such as a glass of warm milk, mild coco or a tea spoonful of honey a cup of camomile tea with a tea spoonful of honey, one other sweet sleep food is a wheat bread honey sandwich which is easy to digest things like a cup of mushroom soup is ideal before bed and it helps to produce good dream

Mushroom is very good for the nervous system, and for the mentality. Also a ripe tomato before bed is very good, things that are hard to digest can some times cause constipation and if it is not identified straight a way it can also cause stress which leads to depression. Constipation is one of the hidden causes of stress if our bowels is not open at least twice a day, we can find our selves with deep depression and cannot find out why because we may have our bowels open once a day

So a lot of orange, tangerine, and funny enough apples and drink a lot of water especially carbonated water that should help the bowels to be more freely and frequent and so help to balance our stress pattern

Another bed time food is bread a good source of vitamin b complex we must not miss out on our vitamin b complex it helps the concentration and help to calm the whole of the body system. It also helps us not to become stressful and helps to deter depression. So wheat bread, brown bread, white bread are equally good

A sandwich of salad, not meat or cheese is well recommended it helps us to have natural dreams that can be define

We should remember not to over indulge in any food whatsoever we should eat just enough that our stomach can hold. You will find that a lot of food that are wholesome for our wellbeing is not mentioned this is to remind that we are vulnerable and is susceptible mistakenness in society, and is to take care of our selves so this book is to help us with the daily task

Part 12

Some of the must foods

Another of the must food is eggs we should never mistook the importance of an egg the chicken is hatched from it so one egg is an whole fowl and we need just one at a time there are so many ways of enjoying an egg and it nutrients, an humlette, scrambled, fried, porch, boiled, or simply waxy

Egg is rich in zinc protein vitamin B egg is a real nerve food it is easy to obtain an egg to think of its use and the benefit we get from egg makes it a must as part of our diet. Apart from those who are definitely allergic to eating eggs

Women who are pregnant should try to eat an egg every day it will not spoil the diet because of its nutritional value eggs vitamin B is so essential, and it an egg sandwich last thing at night gives a restful night sleep, and you will wake up feeling full of vitality because it balances the body system. A duck egg is recommended once a day if you suffer a breakdown.

A pheasant egg was whisk with a tot of brandy in the Victorian days and was given to a first time mother it is said to balance the mother and baby

Another repair food and laughing food is honey. In the case of stress a glass of lemon juice sweetened with a table spoonful of honey will help to calm the nerve and so balance the situation. Honey holds a vase amount of energy and vitamins honey is a cure all and can be use to remedy almost any ailment, it is highly recommended as a night cap if you should have a cup of camomile tea sweetened with a tea spoonful of honey it will assure you of a steady night sleep

Some of us gets a good night sleep yet still wake up in the morning feeling sluggish. Well to have a cup full of any hot drink sweetened with a tea spoonful of honey or enough to your taste will help you to wake up feeling fresh and well rested. Honey is not just a night time food it is also a day time pick me up and is full of energy

There is a way of ensuring you not feeling hungry after the evening meal, and that is to have a bowl full of soup as a snack instead of a sandwich. Soup made with several root vegetable instead of croutons

One of the best soup to have is those that have a sensible amount of oil and fibre, protein, zinc which you get from most vegetables but mostly from lentils. The recipe for this soup is quite simple to make

Get a pound of lentils, or as much lentils as require put a least three table spoonful of olive oil, or rape seed oil in the soup pot with the lentils with the amount of water judging with your instinct from how many the soup is going to feed. Three medium size onions
Two cloves of garlic crush
A hand full of celery
One large leek
One pound of medium ripe tomatoes which must be chopped
A small portion of paprika
A tea spoonful of ground cumin
Three medium size potatoes wash and cut in medium size pieces
A sensible amount of chopped coriander
A small amount of chopped parsley

Eat Yourself Mentally Fit

Soak the lentils for about an hour before you put it to the boil to be cooked after the lentils are cooked you add all the other ingredients and lower the heat that you are cooking on so the in gradients will simmer for at least fifteen minutes while you sprinkle a small amount of course black pepper, and if you have at hand a few sweet chilli peppers chopped nicely and spread over the soup as it simmer. You then serve it as hot as possible with a pinch of sea salt to taste

Some people would like the taste of the ingredients more in the soup so you fry the ingredients apart form the lentils which you cook and this time you add a pinch of salt to the lentils before you add all the other ingredients

Some people love the raw taste of what they are eating such as celery, and coriander to achieve the full taste and hold the value and goodness of whatever you are cooking is to cover the sauce pan and use low fire allowing the ingredients to simmer for about half an hour and don't forget to taste and try the ingredients to ensure that everything is cooked, and that is how you ensure to seal the goodness especially when you are cooking soups

When thing to eat is cook properly it ensures palatable taste, and to do the work it is meant to do, such as driving hunger pangs away and keep you fortified all night through which help the sleeping pattern ensuring a steady nerve that way you do not use up too much energy because you are balance, and so run on the normal amount of energy. It is good to store up energy in case of a crisis you have excess to tap into

Now here is another dinner that will keep you full all through the night giving you a restful night with full sleep. One pound of ox liver slice thin
One large onion or two medium ones chopped nicely
One table spoonful of chopped coriander
One table spoonful of chopped parsley
Three large sweet chilli pepper chopped
One tea spoonful of course black pepper
A pinch of sea salt
One table spoonful of tomato puree
Wash the liver making sure the water is drained off and then flour it to prepare it for frying

Please do not fry dry just fry enough for it to hold the ingredients
Place in a frying pan three table spoonful of olive oil or rape seed oil
Then place the liver into the cold oil on the fire allowing it to sizzle on both sides so you wait for the oil to get heated with the liver in it.

After both sides of the liver is fried you add one tea spoon full of vinegar or a tea spoonful lemon juice on the liver. Add the chopped ingredients on top of the liver with six table spoon full of water then you cover the frying pan on a low flame leave it to cook for 15 minutes and you serve it with mash potato or boil rice, and with one or two tomatoes slice nicely

This one is to help you catch up on your protein keep you full all day long when you eat it for dinner you will forget about feeling hungry at supper.
Half a pound of black eye peas
One lime juice
Two cloves of chopped garlic
Two table spoonful of rape seed oil
The same of olive oil

Eat Yourself Mentally Fit

One table spoonful of tomato puree
Half of tea spoonful of rough black pepper
Two chopped medium onion
One tea spoonful of chopped parsley
One tea spoonful of coriander
Mix the tomato puree with the onions and other ingredients after you bring the black eye peas to the boil, and it is cooked, you use you discretion in cooking the black eye peas you keep it open the flame until they are cooked

Because some peas is harder than some

Sizzle the onion and coriander, parsley, and garlic then you drain the water from the peas leave to dry out for fifteen minutes and then with a pinch of sea salt you mix everything together in the sauce pan after mixing well you leave to simmer you leave for five to ten minutes you serve with mash, or rice you can even have it on toast for supper hoops you add one table spoonful of good butter to the hot cooked ingredients

No one tried nuts and peas well it is highly nutritional it is a blend and makes quite a balance meal.
Half a pound of kidney beans
Half a pound of chopped mix chopped nuts
Boil the kidney beans until it is cooked enough to eat
After the beans are cooked it is important that you put the beans to dry by draining off the water that it is cooked into leaving it to dry for a few minutes mix the cooked beans and the nuts together along with one tea spoonful of cumin seed
Half a tea spoonful of cayenne pepper
Half a tea spoonful of paprika
 A pinch of sea salt
One table spoonful of olive oil butter, or other vegetable oil that is to melt to mix with the rest of the ingredients

Half a pound of chopped tomato
Mix everything together putting one tea spoonful of lemon juice, and one tea spoonful of vinegar any type will do cover and leave to simmer for 15 minutes then serve with rice. These are all filling food that is protein fortified that will keep you feeling fit and full

Here is one for morning time or night time brunch or just as an ordinary snack
3ozs of stone grown wheat flour mix with 2ozs of brown rice flour
3 well beaten eggs
One level tea spoonful of mix spice
3 oz of brown
One lemon rind
3 table spoonful of orange juice
1 lime rind
One table spoonful of lime or lemon juice
Half a pint of milk
Place all the ingredients into a blender for one or two minutes until the mixture is thoroughly blended and mix evenly.
Put a little olive oil or rape seed oil into a prying pan heat it well be sure that the frying pan is non stick
When the pan and the oil is heated pour enough of the mixture to cover all sides of the pan for one or two minutes turn it on the other side for the same period of time remove the pan cake from the frying pan and place it into a warm oven until the rest is cooked

You can fill this pan cake with almost any type of filling. One of the most appropriate is apricot filling

6 to 8 apricots wash and seed dash a pinch of cinnamon and a pinch of nutmeg the juice of two oranges sweetened with a table spoonful of honey mix well then place the apricots into the mixture slowly mix and spoon

Eat Yourself Mentally Fit

into the pancake and then roll using as much of the mixture as needed. Apart from sharran fruit can also be used also pears also sultanas and raisons cherries dates and prunes using the same amount orange juice cinnamon and nutmeg as mentioned

You will find this very delicious and nourishing it is a brilliant breakfast food or last thing at night snack. You may find the amount of rind from the lemon and lime a bit much but the orange juice and the honey mixture compensate to the taste

It is what goodness comes from the ingredients that make this mention a priority full of vitamin b and several of the mineral the body needs. For older people it is a must, and for children because of the taste you will have no problem with them eating and enjoying it. It is full of energy so instead of the oily and starchy snack why not try making the summer jack pancake

You will find that with this pancake you need not drink a lot of fruit juice but plain water that is what you will feel for after eating it which is good it helps the detox process

Here is a recipe for purely stock chicken
It is full of goodness
6 chicken thighs
3 medium tomatoes
Half a pound of chopped Brazil nuts
 One tea spoonful of chopped coriander
One tea spoonful of chopped parsley
3 large chopped onions
2 medium sweet peppers chopped
3 large sweet chilli peppers chopped
1 pint of chicken stock
Brown the chicken thighs

Sizzle the chopped ingredients in four ounces of butter preferable olive butter
Place the chicken along with the ingredients into a sauce pan big enough to hold all of the ingredients, and the stock. Place the chicken firstly in the stock in the sauce pan then place all the chopped ingredients on top of the chicken, cover and leave on low heat to simmer for half an hour it is best to bring every thing to the boil before turning the heat on low flame to simmer

Put a pinch of sea salt in the stock just to blend it after half an hour you can serve it with cuscus or rice. When a meal is cooked with as much vegetable it is not necessary for you to have huge amount of vegetable to accompany the meal one or two is enough unless you are trying to catch up on some vitamin, and minerals

Some times we of to learn to develop a taste for food other than the food we are accustom to. Such as foods from other parts of the world other than from where we are from such as food from the tropics it is as though that extra sunlight and heat does some thing for the food from the tropics. Such as the plantain, dasheen, and the many species of yam, and sweet potatoes, eddoes and green bananas, coco and ackees they are full of goodness. If you are a blood pressure sufferer you should have the amount of these well starched food checked and measure for partaking in them fully.

Things such as sweet cassava which is full of starch, iron, calcium, potassium, and zinc it is very good for the nerve, and is a remedy for stress, but the starch context give cause for concern to blood pressure sufferer

Grater two pounds of sweet cassava, and squeeze it and run it through a sieve bearing in mind that the sweet cassava should be pealed before you grater it you stand

Eat Yourself Mentally Fit

the juice in a bowl for half a day for it to settle and set you then throw off the water that settled on top of the starch it formed you leave it to dry for another half a day scrape from the bowl the substance that will look like wet flour and leave to dry in a open plate you then crush it into a powder

That evidently is the starch of the cassava bearing in mind that there is bitter cassava, and sweet cassava you should never use the bitter cassava for any thing else but medicine for animals. Word had it that test shows that it can be use for human pancreatic treatment but it should not be eaten, but the sweet cassava is only for eating, and so the starch of the sweet cassava can be use for porridge and to thicken gravy. After you make sure that the sweet cassava starch is carefully dried and become a powder you put a pint of milk into sauce pan and bring it to the boil

You then put in it half a tea spoonful of mix spice making sure that one of the spice being nut meg, you stir and put one table spoonful honey and one of glucose sugar you put into a bowl three table spoonful of the sweet cassava starch you add a little water to make a runny paste. While the milk is slowly boiling you pour and stir in the mixture stirring whiskey so it do not form any lump.

Making sure that all the ingredients are mix well together before bringing to the boil so when you add the starch it blends nicely with this you can add one table spoonful of good brandy, if giving to babies you can leave out the brandy. You do not of to leave it for any length of time to boil five minutes will do and stir well

You lift it from the heat or flame and stand it in a cool place and serve at once for the building of the nerve you can also add two table spoonful of buck fast wine or

sanatogen tonic wine after all it is to settle the nerves and without the alcohol feed it
to babies who suffers bad teething and those who are two active to handle

You can also drink the compound mixture warm or with crush ice in many case a pint of Guinness can also be added to the mixture for those who are suffering a breaking and is taking medication it helps a great deal to calm the nerve

This procedure can be use for older people with a threat of forgetfulness this was sworn by the native Australians when ever any one was diagnose mad it calms the sufferer, and lessons the attack

Please bear in mind that the sweet cassava tonic can be made without alcohol and with simple milk, nutmeg, cinnamon and be mix with an infusion of chainie root, and strong bark bring to the b oil for about one hour then stand in a cool place to cool and then strain and mix the mixture with the cassava starch and condense sweet milk and use as a tonic

Bearing in mind that to a pound in weight chainnie root, and the same in strong bark two pints of water is to be poured in a large enough sauce pan and bring to the boil until it is only one pint then you add the milk which should be condense sweet milk to taste with a rich sweet taste by then you would have boil one cup of water and mix the sweet cassava starch in a paste and pour the boil water on it bringing it to one full cup of paste mixture which is thick in texture to add to the other mixture stir well and serve

It is a well known cure for lost of sleep

Eat Yourself Mentally Fit

Many people who are mentally ill is highly over weight, and find it difficult to keep to a even weight well daily intake of vegetable, fruits and measured quantity of root food such as potatoes sweet and other wise with the root vegetables such a Swede, parsnip beet root, carrot and several others that is not easily found in England but is imported and is seasonable base

The root tuber such as yam dasheen cocoas and eddoes, eddoes holds a good amount of zinc, iron, potassium, and oxide not many food contain oxide it also holds a vase amount of vitamin b complex. To liquidise the eddoes after pealing them you put in the frying pan 3 table spoonful of olive oil

Whip an egg with some chopped basil black pepper and fry as you would a fritter making sure that it is turn on both sides and keep on low flame for about ten minutes both sides.

Not only is it tasty it is very nourishing bearing in mind that it is very fattening and should be eaten in small quantity regularly if you feel you are nearing a break down, or if you feel very stress or depress. It is a nerve tonic but should not be fed upon but use as a medicine

Since it cannot be explain why when any one become mentally ill part of the prognosis is the effort to keep at a balance weight we can gain weight eating almost any thing and with the many steroids that can be given for treatment and is known to and is known to be the cause of weight gain. It is important that it is known that all these tonic and suggested foods can cause weight gain if they are not measured in the sense of portions and quantity

It is important to check with a doctor before embarking upon any food or drink for mental stability. Another tonic like drink that is very good for the nerve is the ripe banana and sea mass tonic

3 medium ripe bananas quarter tea spoonful of nutmeg
Half a pound of fresh sea mass
A generous portion of red melon
1 pint of full cream
1 table spoonful of honey
1 table spoonful of glucose
Bring to the boil the sea mass in just over half a pint of water stir until the sea mass is completely dissolve stand in a cool place to cool
Peal the ripe bananas and put it in the blender
Add the cream honey nutmeg and glucose and the melon together blend well and then add the sea mass and then blend again and serve eat like ice cream from a bowl or drink from a glass

If you use the liquid milk this must be taken as a course for a day or two. It can be place in the fridge for the duration of that course

    Whilst the many recipes and advice are being used please bear in mind that many of the items used must be measured because of weight gain if the mentioned food is fed upon frequently without weighing and measuring. There are many food that is good for our mental health that do not threaten weight gain

There are some of them
Cucumber
Celery
Leek
Skimmed milk
Soft cheese

Eat Yourself Mentally Fit

Fish
Chicken
Vegetables

Such as leafy vegetables, the root vegetables such as Swede, parsnip, carrot do come with a limited amount of starch and so should be eaten in limited amount potatoes also should be eaten in recommended amount, or portion that should be eaten

A jacket potato is much healthier to eat to that of a boil, or fried one. Lean meat is recommended and not fatty meat, and a bone soup is recommended but not to be fed on. Only as part of a nourished diet in small quantity

All these advise, is to help prevent what causes stress, depression, and any thing that cause things to play on the mind. Most of all the recommended food helps to strengthen the nerve which is most important, which is why in our daily lives although we may eat the right food some times the food we eat may lack freshness which deter its natural goodness

So to introduce some good supplement especially those with zinc
Iron
Vitamin B complex, protein and calcium which is good with all other compliments are also important to the body but for the mental frame the ones mention is vital

Potato pizza
Two pounds of sweet potato grated
6 table spoon full of olive oil
5 table spoon full of tomato puree
2 cloves of garlic crushed
2 large chopped spring onions
Half a dozen plum tomatoes chopped

One large green pepper chopped
8 ounces of good cheese grated
3 small sprigs of rose marry
A pinch of sea salt
A small amount of course black pepper
Heat the oil into a frying pan adding a little of the potato pressing it into a circle leaving room for it to be turn and cook for 2 to 5 minutes until the base is golden. Turn it over on the other side for to be cooked until it is golden, turn the fritter base on a sheet of baking paper. Cook the remainder using the same method

Mix the tomato puree with the crushed garlic and spread over all the potato base spread it so it cover all the edges spread the spring onion over the bases add the plum tomato and green pepper rose marry and cheese and the salt and pepper
Place the pizza like dress potato under the grill for 7 to 12 minutes or until they are hot and the cheese begin to melt. You then take from under the grill and serve

Part 13

Things we should know about mental illness

There are areas of mental health that food cannot rectify so we must not mistake that fact with trying to keep assertive, and trying to prevent the illness also to stablize our system to keep well all round with just food. We must live right, and try to synchronize our mind with the right thoughts and know how to take care of our nerve not to over task our body.

Those of us who have an heredity to mental health should not rely on just food to heal the illness but try to get good medical treatment, and also counselling. Some times it is by talking that we learn that our illnesses whatever it may be is heredity.

In our lives we should always try to have a thorough check up with a very good doctor that will include family trait in their case study of your history because the illness relating to mental illness is very worrying and can cause stress if it is a family trait. It can cause people with the illness in their family to be left without being married, or even being disqualified for certain type of job if it is not taken care of

Some job question workers medical history must be issued and if it is found out that they have mental illness it could impede their chances

That an individual is any way a sufferer, and have it as a trait, they would not be considered for the job, yet if you should become ill whilst employed I feel sympathy would be on your side

The study into mental health shows that once you are a sufferer you just do not be better, well that carries a great big question sign, which carries several answers such as to what caused the mental illness, and then how to label it

So we should do the part of the illness justice by preparing for its welfare medically, and other wise. To avoid being mentally ill is to strengthen our nervous frame, along with the right frame of mind, and most important food, and not over tasking our body, or our intellect. We can do this by seeing to it that we get enough sleep

Some time it is difficult to cultivate a good sleeping pattern. We should trying exercising at suggested hours of the day. To do exercise in the morning is good it gives our body enough time to correspond with the days need, and to co-inside with our metabolic

Such a pattern can also change moods. So to change a dull, slugglish mood which most of us could develop through lack of sleep and to have a good feeling throughout the day, we should also check our diet to assure our selves of a sound day. Such food is labelled mood food a simple food as onion, and especially red onions and the complete vitamin B complex

Vitamin B complex will assure you of calcium, and assertiveness hence to have a positive out look on the various aspect of life. To be able to control mind over mood is wonderful, because this is where the notice of a diagnosis start. The mood that set you to know that something is not right, most of us do not reflect on our diet, but to get to the doctor

For what the mind tells you waiting for a confirmation, when nine out of ten times the doctor will diagnosis that you are certainly stress or depress and treat you for it. While the medicine works it takes far much longer for you to become well unless you are told by the doctor to start a monitored diet

Which is why in the very near future there will be a diet centre for the mentally ill, so the nerve and the mind can be given prescribed foods which will be a great saving on the NHS because most of those food are cheaper than long term drugs there will be drugs but it will be compensated with prescribed food

Which is why this book is to commence the guide line of the starting point after the counselling and initial drugs, food will be prescribed and with strict order of appliances. Some times we depend only on the drugs and hang up all the know how, well our food is going to become more important

To our every day way of life, because it is the food that sustain us while the drugs repair, and help to maintain in other words control the illness. Mind food is of great importance and it stem from vitamins and minerals, and the every day nourishment that we feed our body, these food can only counteract bad and find there way into doing right for our mind body, and mental stability

Our whole complete frame work and nervous system rely on the right food, rest and a will power to maintain the right mental faculty. In all we do food plays the most important roll

One of the most important mint food is green banana the porridge of the green banana is filled with iron and other minerals one of them being calcium, and the other is protein. It is very important to feed the mind, because the mind is the fundament of our well being

If you can control the mind then you can by pass at of the wear tear of our well being to put our frame work on a more constructive level to maintain a healthy life. The chocho, and cucumber is known to be a mind food as well as the pumpkin and marrow also courgettes. All marrow type foods are highly essential it helps the concentration and the building of the strength to the mental frame to the body.

Most marrow type vegetable is full of vitamin B complex and so it also helps the nervous system

So food such as guillotine and sea moss chicken foot goats foot cows foot pigs trotters are highly recommended nerve food and will help to maintain a good structure to and for our mental frame

One way of assuring our selves of getting the best from those food items that is mentioned is to for instance get one chopped cows foot be sure to have a big enough pot to hold the complete chopped cows foot with a contents of water to full the pot not to the rim but enough too cover the chopped cows foot to withstand the duration of the cooking. Most people use a pressure cooker to cook the cow foot but a pot is just as good but it takes longer to cook using a pot

You add a little sea salt to taste and leave it to cook. You should leave the cows foot to cook for as long as it takes to cook until it is jelly soft. You then lift the meat off the heat and stand it aside to cool so you can separate the bones

Then strain the liquid stand it aside with the jelly looking meat in a bowl get 3 cloves of garlic and crush it along with a generous amount of water cress, and the same of horse radishes and the same of mustard tops with 4 or 5 spring onions, two large red onions a tea spoonful of course black pepper one table spoonful of good vinegar

You chop the spring onions the red onions the water cress the mustard tops along with the garlic and introduce them all to the meat and the juice and then mix by stirring gently to bring all the flavours together you then stand it in a cool place or in the refrigerator until it forms a thick jelly with all the ingredients in it

You serve it in a bowl or if you prefer, with all the ingredients in you can return it to the heat and serve it hot.

Some of us have faith in herbs well there are some herbs that can be sworn by. There are some that have medicinal properties that countries all over use as part of a prescribe method to cure. These herbs that you are about to embark upon has more than one use in the sense of remedy.

Before these herbs are use please quote that to mix you should first seek medical advice from a doctor, a herbalist, or your pharmacist and not to mix them with any medication unless you are adviced to do so by the people mentioned

Some herbs are potent on its own and can be a danger if use with any thing else especially chemicals. So before taking any type of herb please consult your doctor for good result from any herbs unless advise other wise each herb should be used on its own for a complaint, that way you can monitor its potency, because some times the body react to one herb differently to how it react to another

Here are few of the types of herbs and plants you can buy over the counter from any herbalist, to help you to steady the nerve and help you to think positive also to keep you if you are curious to any strangeness of feeling in the way you think or some times even your sleeping pattern may change from an even pattern to a uneven pattern

Even when you are only curious if you are on medication you must contact a qualified herbalist or your family doctor before using any of the following mentioned herbs or plants. Your local chemist is fully qualified to advise you on what you should take and what you should not. Some of us are very reluctant in going into a chemist shop to ask medical question, well it is strongly advisable to go along to a chemist shop to ask advice from a qualified pharmacist

Seeing that we cannot just pop into a doctor's surgery at random many a deaths, and what end up to become chronic complaints could be easily be dwelt with if we would take the initiative to pop into our local chemist to ask medical advice instead of waiting until our feeling become so apparent that when we manage to get to our doctor we are either hospitalise or of to be put on medication, to prevent an illness such as developed stress, depression or nervous disorder which can be caused by a number of slowly developed enigmas

Which if were taken in consideration at an early stage it would have had lesser consequences than being caught when it is already it is already to late these plants are use for other complaints which is why it is best too ask advice of qualified people before attempt using them, because what seems like one complaint may be another but closely link, and required another herb, or plant as a preventative method

Making it plain about the safeness of the remedy and method used in this book is most important so bear with reading about the actualities until we reach the climax of where we can start the names of the actual plants and herbs.

We start with plants the first one is hop, many people see hop as the association with alcohol, well hop can be use as a mild sedative to help us sleep, and also it can be use as a tea to keep us calm. Hop without alcohol is a great beverage it can also be use to regulate the urine

The other is yarrow which can be used as a mild tranquillizer if ever you are feeling highly strong or agitated. An infusion of tea which should be used in small quantity such as about 3grams of the flowers two to three times daily if you are staying at home and is not driving because it causes drowsiness, at the same time it settles you to a restful sleep or calm interval which settles the nerve

Borage is known to calm the nervous system and help to restrain fatigue. It is a plant that has several uses, but especially for the treatment of depression. It bears the same values as evening primrose

Wild strawberries can be use as a tea for nervousness, both the fruit, and the leaves. The fruits can be eaten with discretion, and the leaves 1gram can be used as a tea three times a day until the condition eases

Many of us do not pay attention to tenseness, which it is a growing reason to the development of stress. To help the condition here are some plants that can be use at the consent of a doctor or a qualified herbalist, or pharmacist

Lemon balm or even the common balm can be use to dissolve tenseness and bring you to a calm relax settled mood this plant is also good for nervous exhaustion 3 to 4 grams is recommended as an infusion two or three times a day if you are a mental health sufferer, if you are a new mother this plant do interfere with the production of milk if the new mother is breast feeding, so caution should be taken if this plant infusion is going to be used orally

On a whole this plant is recommended if you have mental fatigue the flower is most potent as a tea it also help you to a restful night

The mint and all its family is a soothing remedy some people thinks that the word peppermint is use only for indigestion or for stomach upset, but the peppermint and the common mint black mint is a good relaxing remedy for mental disorder a strong infusion of two mints mix together will give you a calm mind, and help you to sleep peacefully

Eat Yourself Mentally Fit

It is now known that the peppermint make in strong doses can be used for colonic disorder

It is suspected that if the colon is sick it can cause severe stress which leads to tenseness, so to mix two mints together one of what must be the peppermint will help to control the situation enough to have it repelled. Please bear in mind that there are several species of mints, and all of them all of them is valuable

Wild marjoram known also as oregano this plant is known also as a tranquillizer and also is use to control mood changes. Two grams of this plant should taken twice daily until the situation cleared up, please bear in mind although marjoram is sometimes used in cooking if you are pregnant, or is breast feeding you should not attempt to use this plant orally

Burnet saxifrage is use too help promote a settled mind many of us feel only tablets and counselling can settle the mind, well burnet saxifrage is a tonic that help control feeling, and mood hence help you to think positive. That way you will find that you will be able to deal with tenseness and stress because the mind strengthened with the tea made from burnet saxifrage it is a most powerful plant in an herbal sense

Black currant is some time seen as a tonic for colds and fever, it soothe and relax and can be relied upon to assist in nerve irruption when any one starts to think irritationally a hot cup of black currant with a tea spoonful of lemon juice can help you to stop thinking and instead take a nap

When you are in a temper a cool glass of strong black current will help you to feel rational enough to calm down and discuss instead of prolonging an argument. At night a glass or cup of hot or cold black currant can help you to get a good night sleep. All these issues are made to help the mentally ill, any thing to help calm and control the situation namely the illness is helping to strengthen mental attitude

To eat black current as a fruit if you eat a considerable amount it will put you in a relaxing mood almost like a tranquillizer

Rue is a very important plant it helps to cure nervous head aches which could lead up to an irruption of mental disorder cause by interference of the nerve. Rue helps to control the nerve it helps the rush of blood and so calm the situation so the whole nervous pattern become well and control it also helps vertigo a complaint many mental health sufferer suffer from, because of the balancing although this plant is so very useful any one that is pregnant or breast feeding should not part take of it without medical say so

Small leaves thyme is very good for people who are suffering from nervousness, stage fright and shy a cup of this plant using 4 grams of the flowers or leaves to make a cup of drink before you go on stage or before you meet a group of people, or even before you sit an exam will calm the nerve and settle the anxiety pattern so you will feel safe to carry out the existing task. It is advisable for pregnant mother to seek the advice of a doctor, or a pharmacist or a qualified herbalist before participating in using this or any other herb

Existing breast feeding mothers should also seed medical advice if they are going to use this herb

Eat Yourself Mentally Fit

Oats is well known for making porridge and is also use to make up muesli and oat meal. This precious plant is a tonic in many ways for the nerve, for depression and for insomnia it also helps with the urinary tracts. It helps with the disposal of excess fluids. When convalescence it is especially use to get you back to a normal way of life as possible. The plant supply a great deal of natural substances that helps the debilitated nervous system it also helps as a remedy for exhaustion

Oats acts as a stimulator for the whole complete body system and nervous system because of its strong effect the amount that should be used should be measured the amount of alkaloid in oats make it a most potent tonic which is therapeutic and helps to relax the body system all round. On a whole oats can be used in several ways to a recipe

Caution should be taken when eating because to over indulge could cause severe head ache. Unless you have ways of burning up some of the energy it gives then you should eat only a recommended amount until the situation is cleared up

Depression as we know is the main rout to mental health please do not misconstrued the fact that mental health illness can because from a number of things but nine out of ten cases it always start as a developing trait which grow from stage to stage

As there are many avenues to mental health illness please know that these herbal plants remedies can also help to train the mind to relax, and to help users think positive

These plants are well known and can be bought from any good herbalist

Ladies slippers is a nerve tonic root it helps to calm the nerve relieve tension and rid depression, and after any unhappy mood a cut of the tea can make you become happy again. It is even good for head aches and anxiety it is a panacea to nervous disorder it should be taken for a complaint, and not to be taken at random

Passion flower is use as a tranquillizer it also helps to relax the nervous system and help individual to sleep well at night

This could well become a depended upon herb, so users are warned to be sure that they do not over indulge. Hence why users are ask to submit to a qualified herbalist the reason for taking it

It is not dangerous, but because it relaxes you so much it could become depended upon yet you could not become addicted to it

Cowslip for giving restful sleep it also help to heal nervous tension and is especially known to cure arthritis. Cowslip has wide range of medical usefulness but because this is to advice and help mentally ill people it is mainly issued on the use for tension, depression, anxiety and stress

Anemone known as meadow anemone or pasque flower and is known to relieve nervous tension situation and is a great help in treating neuralgia. It helps to calm you if you are feeling irritable people in Greece usually call it calming plant.

Iris moss is a nerve food, and tonic for the nervous system. It is very thick which many people use as a thickening agent for soups and gravy

Eat Yourself Mentally Fit

Iris moss is an exceptionally nourishing food which is rich in vitamin B complex. It can be use as porridge with milk and nutmeg and sugar preferable brown sugar or glucose.

Wild cherry is another of the panacea plant it helps those who are suffering from nervous cough. It settles irritation, and anxiety it has several other use you can learn of from a herbalist, or a pharmacist

Raspberry is high inn iron and is recommended as part of a control diet because it can be bought all year round it is one of the panacea remedy with so many different use. Let us stick to the main reason of this book and if you should develop a malady you seek the advice of you doctor, pharmacist, or herbalist

Do remember this is just one species of raspberry there are others that are cultivated for eating with the same medicinal properties and which is filled with vitamins and minerals

120 here are some very important herbs that carry vitamin b complex which is so very essential for our mental stability
Water cress B2
mustard seed B2
Kelp B1, B2, B12
    Comfrey B12

Here are some very special fruits that have some essential vitamin such as raspberry, elder berries, rosehip we should try as much as possible never to go without these berries

Please quote that these fruits and vegetables that are mentioned have other vitamins and minerals than the ones mentioned in this book this book is to help you choose the right ones for mental health problems. Eating or using these will give you other worthwhile benefits also

Let me mention again our body needs all known beneficial vitamins and minerals to ensure us of a healthy lifestyle. To k now which of them carries the properties that is beneficial to our mental is what this book is about, there are other books that will give you a round up of the body needs in general

The simple water cress is so beneficial to our health it high in calcium, folic acid, vitamin A, vitamin B2, and vitamin C it is a must on our plate

It is good to know what is good to tone up the whole complete body, and especially the bone. When the bones are well it helps to strengthen the rest of the body, at least you can rely on that area of the body to sustain the frame work of the body

Here are just few of the herbs that is considered good for the muscles and the bones
Comfrey
Horse tail
These two are very good for relaxation and have silica which is essential for all the active bones they strengthen the formation, and the elasticity of the component of the joints
Kelp and alfalfa give a complete range of vitamins and elemental traces of needed vitamins, and minerals for the repair of the bones and muscle

These are also known remedies for relaxation

Cramp bark

Valerian
Skullcap
These help relaxes and tone the nerves muscles up. This book explains a lot about nerve please do not think for one minute that all mental cases starts from the nerve some times the brain and min d has every thing to do with the cause of the mental illness, but the most common traits is the nerve so we deal with this area first

Not forgetting that all that is recommended by way of advice is of the body system
Wolly fox gloves is also good for the relief of stress and pressure in any way, pressure at work a cup of foxgloves before retiring to bed at night will assure you of a morning awakening full of vitality, and ready for the day a head. It is widely used for the strengthening of the blood vessels it is often time use in the accompanying with other herbs by qualified herbalist.
Eyebright is use for distension and hallucination, and also can help strengthen the mind, hence help you to think straight and correctively. It can also be used as a treatment to lower high blood pressure, please do not use it if you are pregnant or breast feeding

You will find that most of the ideas given in the recipes have no specific cooking time it is because the book is aimed at strengthening the reader independence and to help balance the sense of knowing that every one can cook to an extent. Most mentally ill people have a very high I Q and need to keep it that way and to be able to maintain it

So to give people a reason to use their intelligence is good especially when if one is diagnose mentally ill, the first area of their handicap is their intelligence, and then their independence

You can reach from step to step by asking question on how long things takes to cook, things such as a potato you would put to the boil and because salt is not an essential to some people but will not do any harm if you did use a little to cook a potato some people would say it is very easy to cook

To cook potatoes you could put the amount you require into a pot with enough water to cover them putting a small amount of salt into the water then leave it to cook on an understandable gas mark, or electric in mentioning this I am not robbing you, or invading your intelligence

Many people thinks that if someone is manic depress, or vaguely mentally ill they have lost every ting but it is not so. Many of us are mentally but still have our intelligence about us. That is because there are many areas, and stages of mental illnesses

To cook vegetables is of the likeliness, and of individual taste some people's vegetables of to be well cooked, while some others of to be just partially cooked it is a matter of preference. Many mentally ill people have a family to cater for and they of to use their intelligence in their likes, and dislikes in food. So to leave the cooking instructions to have them use their intellect is actually helping them, that way every thing is not taken away from them instead part of their independence is for them to use their intelligence.

This is what the book is all about to feed individuals with the right food, and the right attitude towards being able to get counted, also with some right attitudes towards their humanity. We eat and now we must drink, drinks are most important to our lives especially drinks that helps us nutritionally. Such as carrot juice, beetroot juice, tomato juice, water cress juice, parsnip juice, and most of all no one knew how important winter cabbage juice was until it was tested first thing in the morning and how it help the person through out the day

Radish juice, and spring green juice, pumpkin juice, Chinese chow juice, and with all of these juice you should try just a little nutmeg the powder or the tincture

To cook yam, dashene, sweet potato, or pumpkin is the same procedure as you would a potato.

Part 14

About our Salt and Sugar intake

Come on let us experiment, put the pot on with enough water to cover the food when you put it into the pot. Many of us do not use salt, but some of us will still have a taste for the spice salt, and should not give it up all together, but lower, or lesson the intake by at least half the normal intake that way you will be on the right tract with the salt intake

Many people will advice you to take no salt whatsoever, I feel that is wrong the body do need certain amount of salt for us to function in a balance way. On like sugar we eat ready make sugar in almost everything we eat now a days, so the made up sugar is not altogether necessary even though it is only the assumption of some people

Some people do of to have some form of sugar as a daily intake to balance the blood sugar level, or they may become ill feeling low, and lethargic and until they have some form of sugar intake they will not feel well. So a little of everything is better for the body than none at all

Now back to how to cook a potato it is quite simple but for those of us who do not know how to cook it could prove a problem. As we all know that the water in any pot with food in it must be boiling in a bubbley way for a while before we can assume that the food in the pot is cooked. One way of knowing whether the food is cook or not is to use a fork and try to take a piece of the food on it, and taste it to be sure that the food is cooked

Eat Yourself Mentally Fit

Another way to be sure that the food is cooked, is after you have found out how long a certain type of food takes to cook, you time it your self and that way you would have done the whole complete cooking all by yourself. I do not think there is any one who has never cook a potato in their whole entire life, if there are any one then let us start from scratch now. Cooking can be such fun especially when it is for such a good purpose as keeping mentally fit.

To cook for your mental health is not only bossing the prestige it strengthens the independence and gives a sense of confidence. After any one is labelled mentally ill they some times feel it is the end of the world for them, well it is not the end of the world it is just the beginning of a new chapter in life one that needs all the co-ordination you can get hold of.

The best way to help yourself when you are mentally ill is to prepare some thing to eat, so you can determine the taste and your likes, and dislikes for the various foods. Bearing in mind that nine out of ten times no one is that far gone that they cannot prepare a meal for them self. If you are part of a get well again programme in a therapeutic way the best thing to do is to do things for yourself, starting by cooking for yourself, taking care of your clothe, abode, and shopping.

All these task will help any one who is mentally ill to get back to reality and to appreciate themselves again, which is why to dress your self with your own opinion, and to cook something to suite your taste is always the right thing to do. As a measure and cooking as a part of your independence is good because someone may say you should put a tea spoon of salt, but it is you who taste the cooking and know that half a teaspoonful will do just as good, in saying so to develop a taste for less salt is a very good thing.

Many of us cook with more seasoning to avoid using the excess salt, so it is a matter of taste where salt is concern. If the meat is cooked with salt then there is no need for the vegetables or the food such as rice, pasta, potatoes, or cuscus to be cooked with salt because the gravy or just the meat will contras the taste and will balance the salt context.

One way of rectifying our salt intake is to find out how much salt the body needs in a day then check carefully the food we eat each day to find out whether it is already made up with salt so we do not eat over the amount we should really have. We should carry out the same procedure with sugar with an exception to those of us who has to have sugar as part of their surviving kit.